BIG BAD ASS

· BOOK OF ·

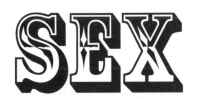

Nancy Armstrong

STERLING
New York

STERLING
New York

An Imprint of Sterling Publishing
387 Park Avenue South
New York, NY 10016

ISBN 978-1-4027-4787-8

Library of Congress Cataloging-in-Publication Data
Armstrong, Nancy, 1976-
  Big bad ass book of sex / Nancy Armstrong.
     p. cm.
   ISBN 978-1-4027-4787-8 (pbk.)
  1. Sex instruction. 2. Sexual intercourse. 3. Sexual excitement. I. Title.
HQ31.A66 2014
613.9071--dc23
                          2014001416

Distributed in Canada by Sterling Publishing
      ℅ Canadian Manda Group, 165 Dufferin Street
           Toronto, Ontario, Canada M6K 3H6
Distributed in the United Kingdom by GMC Distribution Services
Castle Place, 166 High Street, Lewes, East Sussex, England BN7 1XU
Distributed in Australia by Capricorn Link (Australia) Pty. Ltd.
       P.O. Box 704, Windsor, NSW 2756, Australia

            Designed by Philip Buchanan
            Interior art @Shutterstock.com

For information about custom editions, special sales, premium and corporate purchases,
please contact Sterling Special Sales Department at 800-805-5489
or specialsales@sterlingpublishing.com.

Manufactured in Canada

2 4 6 8 10 9 7 5 3 1

www.sterlingpublishing.com

Dedication

*For Keimay, who had a great sense of humor about sex—
and everything else.*

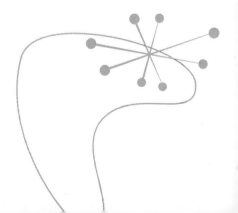

Contents

Part 2: Duets

Stories

Part 3: Three's Company

Stories

Part 4: A Swingin' Party

Stories

Part 5: Extreme Kink

Stories

Introduction:
Making the World Go

Sex is like air:
It's no big deal unless
you aren't getting any.

—Unknown

With all due respect to whoever first coined the phrase, it isn't love that makes the world go round, it's sex. Think about it. (Like you're ever *not* thinking about it!) Without sex, there'd be no kissing, no orgasms, no new life on the planet, no suggestive jokes on television—the list goes on and on. So in a sense, even if it's not responsible for the actual turning of the planet on its axis, sex does make the world *go*. And it's literally everywhere, not just in your bedroom or hot tub or kitchen or tree house: it's pervasive in just about every form of entertainment out there; its influence is reaching kids sooner than it ever has; and as much as they try to keep it out, sex is all over the workplace, too.

So don't you think you'd better have some idea how to do it? Honestly, sex has evolved as quickly as people have in the twenty-first century. It was probably never as cut and dried as some people would have you believe—surely not too many people still subscribe to the in-out-repeat school of coitus—but these days, there are as many ways to do it as there are ways to order coffee (and as many accoutrements, too!). So here we're presenting some basic information, answering questions, giving you tips for how to get it on in style, and even providing some erotic fiction to inspire you to even greater sexual heights.

We've broken things down into five parts:

* **Part 1:** Solo Sex (masturbation)
* **Part 2:** Duets (one-on-one sex)
* **Part 3:** Three's Company (threesomes)
* **Part 4:** A Swingin' Party (group sex)
* **Part 5:** Extreme Kink (the stuff that's weird to 99 percent of the population).

Remember, as Woody Allen once said, "Love is the answer, but while you're waiting for the answer, sex raises some pretty interesting questions." We aim to answer some of those questions in this book.

For those of you who think you already know it all—ha! You couldn't possibly. There's bound to be something in here you never knew or something you never even thought to ask! This book really does have it all; just look how long it is! In these pages, you'll find a veritable smorgasbord of sexual information: everything from masturbating in the shower to handcuffing your lover to the radiator and all the delightful stuff in between. In addition to basic principles of sexuality and ideas and tips for practical use, we've included some motivational erotica at the end of each section, also grouped by subject. Think of the stories as illustrations of the principles you've just studied. (Yeah, *that's* what they are.)

Whether you're interested in heightening your own pleasure with your partner of twenty-five years or getting a person you've known for twenty-five minutes to agree to dress up as an exterminator and spray you with insecticide, this is your guide. There's always more to learn about the world's favorite subject.

ASSORTED DISCLAIMERS

Although there are jokes throughout this book about any number of sexual situations and inclinations, we mean to go at this in a way that is open-minded and not judge anyone's preferences or predilections. As long as no one gets hurt who doesn't want to, it's okay by us.

As you read through this menu of delights, you may notice that there are more "every woman is different" caveats than there are "every man is different" warnings. That's because the mechanics for men are basically the same, whereas women experience orgasms in a couple of different ways. That doesn't mean that all men like the same things, and it doesn't always mean that women are more complicated than men or that something that got one woman off won't work with another.

It's important to remember as you read that every person is different both anatomically and in what turns him or her on. This also means that the fact that something works with one partner or group doesn't mean that it will work with another. Explore. Ask. That's the fun of it.

The stories in this book are meant as fantasies to get you off. They are not necessarily how-to guides. For instance, we demand that you practice safe sex, especially as you add more and more people to the scenario; however, in many of the stories, semen is flying everywhere and the characters aren't always being as careful as they should.

Please, approach everything in this book (or at least everything you choose to approach in this book) with a healthy sense of humor . . . and hygiene.

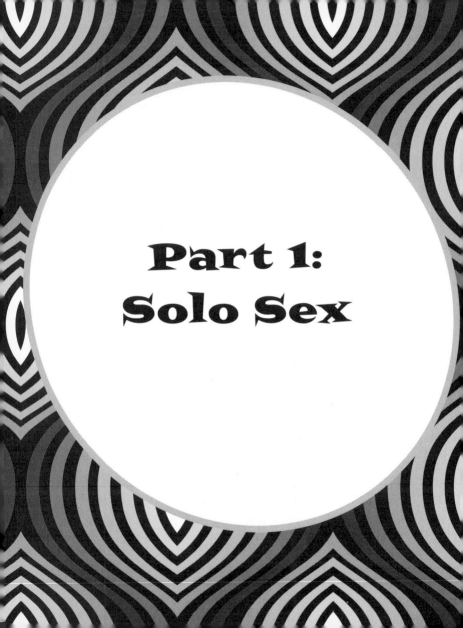

Part 1:
Solo Sex

Don't knock masturbation—
it's sex with someone I love.
—Woody Allen

In general, folks get pretty embarrassed when the topic of solo sex play comes up. For whatever reason, although touching yourself is possibly the most natural, normal thing you can do, there has been a stigma attached to masturbation for as long as most people can remember. In the 1800s, it was widely believed that touching your own sex organs damaged your health, and most of Western civilization is familiar with Sigmund Freud's theories regarding the stages of sexual development: he thought that masturbation was child's play and that if people continued touching themselves into adulthood, their development would be stunted somehow. If you ask a random sampling of your acquaintances about their masturbatory history, in addition to the several slaps and guffaws you're likely to get, you'll probably encounter blushing, guilty faces, and denials aplenty.

BARE FACTS

Masturbation, strictly speaking, is the act of touching oneself sexually to achieve heightened pleasure or orgasm. It's been called any number of things down through the ages, but most of the nicknames refer to what men do with their penises when they're alone: choking the chicken, jerking off, beating the meat, spanking the monkey, and on and on. For women, the euphemisms aren't nearly as colorful—or as violent: fingering, petting the kitty, diddling, and so on. Regardless of what you call it, though, it's fun, free, and harmless to yourself and others. How many things in this world can we say that about?

As far as stats on who masturbates, there's no authoritative number, largely because of the embarrassment factor, but it's safe to assume that in this day and age, most people have fiddled around with themselves at least a little bit. And why not? Touch is the first sense we develop as human beings, and touching ourselves just feels good. Mae West said, "An orgasm a day keeps the doctor away," but what if you're single? Or involved but unable to come with a partner? Or bored? Or having trouble sleeping? According to conventional wisdom, simply wank away. Plus, how will you ever know what you like (and be able to tell someone else) if you don't experiment a little?

SNAP OF THE FINGER

Forget the Ambien. In addition to the pleasure derived from masturbation, it's a natural sleep aid.

Whether you're a boy or a girl, strip off your clothes, get a mirror or stand or sit near one, and take a good look at yourself. There's nothing gross or icky about your own parts—they came with your body and can do some amazing things, including give you (and perhaps others) intense pleasure. But before we get to the—ahem—meat of things, a quick rundown of the equipment.

MEN'S EROGENOUS ZONES

There are all sorts of areas on a man's body that are nice to stroke and kiss, but when he's playing with himself, here's where his attention will usually be focused:

* The *penis* is the main one, obviously, and in general it doesn't have to be treated delicately. Most men touch themselves roughly (as evidenced on page 5 in the list of popular nicknames for male masturbation). The *frenulum* is particularly sensitive; it's the area right under the head on the underside.
* Some men's *nipples* are very sensitive, and some aren't. It will be delightful to figure out your own sensitivity.
* Lots of men like their *testicles* played with, and lots play with their own whenever they get the chance.
* The *perineum* is the strip of skin between the scrotum and the anus, and it may be nice to touch. It also may be ticklish.
* Some men may like a finger in the *anus*; some may not. Some *really* may not.
* Stroking an *inner thigh* may intensify good feelings for a man.

WOMEN'S EROGENOUS ZONES

A woman's body is a veritable minefield of fun spots to touch and tickle. She'll probably concentrate her energies on these parts when she's doing herself, though:

* The *clitoris* is at the top of the vulva and is the only piece of human anatomy—male or female—whose purpose is purely for pleasure. So use it! Women are pretty different when it comes to how hard or soft they can stand to be touched here, so start slowly.
* Lots of women tug or rub their *nipples* while masturbating.
* The statistics are all over the place regarding whether women's orgasms originate in the *vagina* or elsewhere. We say, Who cares? If you like touching yours or inserting a finger or toy while pleasing yourself, go for it. The *G-spot* is just inside the vagina, at the top, and some women claim that orgasms originating there are the most intense.

* The *labia majora and minora* (the outer and inner lips of the vulva) are sensitive areas for a lot of women. Some stroke or pull on them while masturbating.
* The *perineum* is the strip of skin between the vagina and the anus and is highly sensitive.
* Whether she likes a finger or toy in her *anus* is a very personal choice each woman must make for herself.
* A woman may stroke her *inner thigh* sometimes while she gets herself off.

Finally, perhaps the most important erogenous zone for men and women is . . . the *brain*! That's right, if the old noggin's not into it, nothing else will be either. It is very important not to discount the importance of thoughts and feelings as they relate to sex and orgasms and all that good stuff. Granted, you might not always be thinking about them when you come, but what goes on in your brain has the ability to heighten or lessen every sexual experience you have whether you're by yourself or with another person or several. Use it!

STRETCHING THE TRUTH

There is a road in Wales called Cae Onan, which translates to "Masturbation Meadow." Citizens there are petitioning the town council to change the name; though they admit it's sort of amusing, mostly they are—you guessed it—embarrassed.

TOUCHING YOURSELF: A PRIMER

Some people start touching themselves when they're little kids, figure out what they like early, and keep up a healthy exploration of their sexuality throughout their lives, with no one telling them that they shouldn't masturbate or that touching themselves is wrong or bad for any reason. Lucky folks. There are a whole lot of people, however, who for whatever reason are uncomfortable touching themselves at all or even broaching the subject of masturbation. This can be for all kinds of reasons, from prohibitive parents, to religious teachings, to unfamiliarity with their own bodies, to abuse, or it can be for no discernible reason at all. Whatever the case, getting familiar with your own body and what feels good to you is a beneficial exercise regardless of your age or level of experience, sexual or otherwise. Here are some tips for getting acquainted—or reacquainted, as the case may be—with that most useful and arguably most fun personal asset: your body.

LISTEN UP, THIS IS IMPORTANT

Although most modern religions consider masturbation a sin, the Hebrew and Christian bibles are completely silent on the matter. And if you're considering committing some sort of depraved act and masturbation will keep you from doing anything stupid, some Islam teachings say you should go for it.

1. Make sure you are in a place where you feel comfortable, with a privacy level that encourages you to be uninhibited and free. You might try your bedroom or bathroom with the door locked or do it when no one else is home. Also, give yourself enough time to

really get in touch with yourself; you should allow at least an hour for this, if not more. There is no rush when you're learning what you like (though you may feel a certain urgency as you get going).

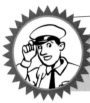

YOU'RE WELCOME FOR THE TIP

If you don't live alone, coordinate everyone's calendar before settling in for some self-loving.

2. Adjust the lighting so that it is not too harsh. A bedside lamp or candle is probably preferable to an overhead light or spotlight. Adjust the temperature in the room so that you will be comfortable completely naked. (Oh, yeah, you're getting totally nude for this exercise. It's required.) Keep in mind that once your blood gets going, you may get a bit overheated. That's fine—and even encouraged!

3. Strip. Take off everything. Do it.

4. If you like, get in a warm bath or hot shower or under the covers. Whatever makes you feel the most relaxed is what you should do.

5. Once you're comfortable in your preferred place, start with some really deep breathing. Try breathing in while counting slowly from one to ten and then exhaling while counting back from ten. Do this several times—though not to the point of light-headedness. The objective is to be relaxed, not breathless (yet).

6. You may fantasize or not while you do this exercise. It's up to you. You will want to concentrate at certain points to see what feels good to you, though, so don't feel that you have to strictly stick to your fantasy.

7. Start by stroking your arms and belly, maybe, or running your fingers up your sides or through your hair. Don't go straight for your genitals; warm yourself up a bit first. Focus on other body parts for several minutes before moving on.

8. Touch your nipples. Try pulling on them or rubbing them in a circular motion. You might lick your fingers before you touch your nipples or try some other form of lubrication. (Further discussion of lube can be found in the next section.)

9a. **Men:** Some men swear by lube; others never use it. It's up to you, but this is the point at which you ought to decide. Once you've taken some time with your nipples, move to your penis and testicles. Grasp the shaft and stroke in an up-and-down motion with a slightly loose fist. Start slowly and work up speed. Tug on your scrotum; run a finger up your perineum; rub against a pillow, a towel, or your mattress. If you like, touch your anus a bit. Do everything slowly at first, until it feels as though you need to speed up. Then do so. Continue doing whatever feels good to you until you can't stand it anymore and then let yourself go. Some men keep stroking themselves through orgasm, and some stop when they start to ejaculate. You can do whatever feels good to you. That's the beauty of being alone.

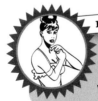

BARE FACTS

Make your own rules as you practice, the only tried-and-true rule being to ride it out in whatever way feels best.

9b. **Women:** Use some lubrication on your fingers. Your own Mother Nature–provided wetness is fine, or it can be saliva if you're not quite there yet. Run your fingers lightly all over your vulva—touch both sets of lips, run your fingers through your pubic hair (if you have any), tweak your clitoris, slip a finger or two inside your vagina. Let your hands travel up and down your inner thighs, keep working on your nipples, and run a finger around your clitoris. Keep it slow in the beginning. When you feel that you must go faster, do so. Keep doing what feels good until the pressure builds to the point where you let yourself go over the edge and have an orgasm. Keep stroking or stop and just press the area around your clitoris.

SECRET TIP

Lots of people have a favorite position when it comes to sex—with or without a partner. Common masturbatory positions for a woman include lying on her back, lying on her stomach with a pillow between her legs, sitting in a chair facing forward or backward, and sitting on top of the washing machine with it set to the spin cycle. Common positions for men include the same, but instead of sitting on the washing machine, a man might stand up in the shower and spank it. Try a few and see what works for you.

LUBRICATION: SLIP N' SLIDE

A question that might arise at this point concerns the best way to get nice and slippery for your solo adventure, assuming your own natural juices aren't giving you quite enough glide. Keep in mind here that lubrication comes in many different types and that lubes that are good for alone time are not always so great for sex with a partner (especially if condoms are involved). So this is a guide to lube for masturbation *only*. Refer to the lubrication sections in the following parts when you're ready to move on to slippery partners.

The best lube for most sex, solo or otherwise, is the water-based kind, of which K-Y® is probably the most famous. There are a slew of types these days—ones that warm up and ones that tingle and anything else you can think of. You can buy lubrication just about anywhere, from the drugstore to the truck stop, so there's no excuse not to have some when you need it. Astroglide® is also very popular.

SNAP OF THE FINGER

Your own saliva is also effective as a lubricant. If you think it's gross to use your spit for sex, you don't have to, but keep in mind that what you're doing is pretty personal, and definitely all natural, and saliva is, in fact, all natural. It's also always available unless it's the morning after a wild and crazy night and you have a mean case of cotton mouth.

When you're getting yourself off and you're a man, you can use any number of household products to grease your path, as it were. Any kind of vegetable oil works just fine, as does baby oil or mineral oil, hand lotion, and Vaseline®, but these are very messy and, depending on the product, might irritate your skin.

For women, the household products that can be used are somewhat more limited, because they can get in and harm the delicate balance that exists inside their vaginas, causing possible infections. A lot of water-based lubes aren't good for the ladies, either, because they contain glycerin, a form of sugar that can cause yeast infections.

A popular type of lube that's on the rise, so to speak, is silicone-based. It is latex-free and seems to keep its slipperiness longer than do other kinds of lube.

However you decide to augment the lubrication Mother Nature has provided for you, keep in mind that lubes designed for sex are the best for sex, and you should check into anything you intend to put on or in your body. Read the labels.

BENEFITS OF MASTURBATION

At this point, you may be asking yourself, Yeah, well, what's so great about masturbation? I have a lover; I don't *need* to get myself off. The simple answer is, good for you.

The slightly longer, more interesting answer for the more thoughtful person is this: touching yourself isn't just a fun time had by all involved. It gives you specific time in which to be with just yourself and learn about your own response. It's also a great way to figure out what you like when it comes to sex with a partner. Heck, failing all that, it's a pretty great cure for insomnia.

Masturbating may help a man control his response when he's with a partner. He may be able to last longer or come more quickly if length of intercourse is an issue with his partner. Touching herself may make a woman more comfortable letting go, making it easier for her to achieve orgasm with or without a partner. And for both men and women, it'll teach them how to teach another person how to touch them in a way that feels splendid.

DANGER

Autoerotic asphyxiation occurs when a person deliberately restricts his or her own breathing right before or during orgasm while masturbating. Whether the heightened arousal comes from the danger of losing consciousness as a result of being unable to breathe or from actually being short of breath is unclear, but either way, this is a bad idea. It is safe to say that as you approach orgasm, you may not be thinking terribly clearly, and it is very unsafe to try to limit a bodily process that literally keeps you alive—at any time and certainly on the mind-blowing road to orgasm. Don't do it.

Self-bondage while masturbating is also not the smartest move unless you are absolutely certain someone will find you quickly should you be unable to loosen your self-imposed restraints. As the name implies, this is when a person ties himself or herself up when going solo. It is often combined with autoerotic asphyxiation, and the two together have caused more than a few experimenters' untimely demise. We're all for ingenuity and imagination when it comes to playing around with solo sex, but these practices are too dangerous for us to endorse. Play it safe and steer clear of them.

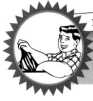

When it comes to helping your masturbatory life grow and evolve, fantasies are the best nutrient.

FANTASIES

As far as guidelines for your fantasy life, there aren't any. Fantasies are just that: fantasy. There is no reason to limit yourself to things that could actually happen, because in most cases, what happens in your fantasies will stay there forever.

So no matter how weird or outlandish or violent or potentially embarrassing your fantasies seem to you, you needn't be ashamed of them or worry about what they say about you or your sexuality. The only point at which you need to rethink this is if you're considering making one of your fantasies a reality or want to share the intimate details of your favorite wank scenario with another person.

This is where things get slightly more complicated. Generally what goes on in people's minds while they touch themselves stays in their minds, and they are content to have fantasies remain fantasies. This is the spirit in which fantasy sharing should be approached. Of course, if you're content to keep your masturbatory fantasies to yourself, that's your prerogative, and it should be respected.

If your wife blurts out that she was thinking about riding a dog naked while you two were making love, do not be too alarmed—or judgmental, either. This doesn't mean she wants to raid the local pet store or that you should call the ASPCA because your neighbor's Pekingese is in danger. It means that one time (or more than once), it may have crossed her mind that something seemingly dirty or decidedly out of the ordinary was kind of hot and got her off.

If you are thinking about actually acting on a fantasy, a bit more caution should be taken. Things such as safety, comfort level, and all parties' acquiescence should be at the top of your essentials list for acting out a fantasy. Under no circumstances should any fantasy that is dangerous to or against the will of any involved party be attempted. More discussion of specific fantasies comes later in this book, so look there for other lists of essential items in fantasy play (bondage, role playing, domination, threesomes, swinging, etc.).

PORN SCORN?

Visual and written representations of sexual congress have been around practically since the beginning of time. From the ancient Romans to the *Kama Sutra* to Victorian smutty novels (everyone needs a good rogering!), our forefathers enjoyed looking at or reading about lusty scenarios. And we still do. Whether you prefer *Penthouse* or *Playgirl*, erotic stories like those found in this book, good old-fashioned VHS/DVD porn, or any of millions of Internet sites devoted to every aspect of sex you can think of (and some you probably never wanted to), there's something scintillating for everyone. And everyone has his or her opinion on what porn is and isn't. But for our purposes, we're talking about any written or visual display that's meant to titillate and excite people in a sexual way.

SECRETS TO MAKE YOU LOOK GOOD

If Internet porn is your thing but you share your computer with others, consider using the Google Chrome browser's Incognito function. The pages viewed with Incognito don't appear in your browser history or search history, and they don't leave cookies on your computer. This lets you enjoy the action without worrying about anyone in your home mistakenly clicking on sluttychix.com.

Probably the main reason most people enjoy erotica and pornography is that these things provide inspiration for getting themselves off while they're alone. (It might be fun to share with a loved one, too, but that's something for the next section.) This is a fine thing to do; there is nothing to be ashamed of, although folks seem to learn as soon as they find out about porn that it should be hidden. The stigma against porn is probably rivaled only by the stigma attached to masturbating at all, so it stands to reason that porn is looked at as something shameful or dirty. (And some of it is.) But pornography and erotica can, in general, serve an important purpose in sexual development.

These titillating displays can help us learn about what turns us on and what doesn't and also provide an outlet for us to vicariously live out fantasies that we wouldn't actually want to experience. The trouble with porn arises when it takes the place of interactions with others or becomes an obsession or addiction. It's also not the best standard (an understatement) to follow when you're looking to learn about how to have a healthy, equal, honest relationship—if anyone goes to porn for that. But as a masturbatory aid, fantasy visualizer, or sexual experimenting device, it's just fine.

TOY BOX

Once you've become comfy with your body and touching it all over and making yourself feel good in ways you may not have before (and you're wondering why you haven't *always* been doing this fun, free, *really fun* activity), you may want to branch out and try some other exciting ways to entertain yourself. In other words, you may enjoy using some props to enhance the experience.

Here's some fun stuff you won't find at the usual toy store, stuff that's meant for adults only, but it's way more amusing than Barbie dolls or LEGOs. (Well, fun in a different way, anyway. We hope.)

First up, *vibrators*. These are objects that require batteries or electricity, which makes them buzz and feel good around or inside your genitals. Generally women use them, but men sometimes may like a little vibe in the butt or buzzing around the balls. They come in so many different forms and shapes and sizes, there's literally a type for everyone. Some are small and mainly for use on and around the clitoris, and others are more penis-shaped and meant for insertion into the vagina. Still others have a piece that goes into the vagina and another piece that buzzes around the clitoris at the same time. Another fun kind has a penislike part for the vagina and a smaller part for the anus. Pretty much if you can imagine it, a sex shop or online store will have it. Go wild!

Next, *dildos*. These are generally penis-shaped and are used by men and women, straight and gay. Unlike vibrators, they don't require batteries or electricity, so they are safe for shower or bath play, and like vibrators, they are made in so many shapes and sizes that it would be impossible to list them all here. They generally are meant for insertion into the vagina or anus, and some are double-headed, some can be strapped on (hence the name strap-on), and some have a suction cup at the end so that you can affix them to a surface for hands-free (or hands-otherwise-occupied) entertainment.

Shower heads, hot tub jets, and *water streams* make good masturbation enhancements as well. Just be careful not to shoot a fast stream of water directly into a woman's vagina, because that can be dangerous.

If a man wants to simulate having sex with a woman, he might try a *pocket pussy*, which is just what it sounds like, though it looks kind of gross. The more expensive they are, the more lifelike they feel, according to unconventional wisdom.

Some men may want to prolong an erection as they masturbate, and that's what a *cock ring* is for. Some models have attachments and protruding bits that are for stimulating a partner's clitoris, but they generally are not used for masturbatory purposes.

Butt plugs are toys that may be used in masturbation, although they are probably more commonly used in anal exploration among couples, because their usual purpose is to keep the anus dilated, or stretched, so that a penis or dildo can go in a bit more easily. Still, some folks may like the feeling of fullness in the anus while they play with themselves.

Other props might come into play during masturbation, such as bottles or rubber gloves or even food. Literally everything under the sun probably has been used in sex play, and we just can't list all of it. But use your common sense and be safe about what you experiment with in the realm of toys and props for masturbation. A good rule of thumb is that if you wouldn't want it in your mouth, don't put it near your private parts either.

YOU'RE WELCOME FOR THE TIP

Recently, there has been a development in the world of sex toys that's cause for celebration. Sex toy parties—in which a salesperson comes to your home with samples and demonstrations and you can buy whatever items you want in relative privacy—have really taken off in the last few years, much to the delight of women everywhere. Called Fuckerware or Passion Parties, they work much like the Tupperware parties of yore: a group of friends (generally women) get together in someone's home, and a representative comes over with a box o' fun and shows the goods. Then everyone can go into a separate room and buy whatever he or she wants from the representative, away from the prying eyes of the other partygoers. These parties are tons of fun and can be very useful, especially if you are embarrassed to go to that XXX sex shop out on the edge of town.

BRING A FRIEND

Although masturbation is very much a solo sport, lots of folks like to practice mutual masturbation, which consists of touching yourself in the presence of another person who is touching himself or herself. Sometimes the participants also may touch each other. This may be done as part of foreplay, or it may be the main course. Either way, it can be very pleasurable and a great way to learn about your own and another person's turn-ons or turn-offs.

You might be asking, Well, if you've got another person to be naked with, why wouldn't you just have intercourse? A reasonable question, assuming that intercourse is always the goal and that all parties emerge from it feeling sexually fulfilled and happy. Sometimes you may not feel like "going all the way" or may want to really explore touching and what feels good to you and your partner in terms of "hands-on" attention. It's a good experiment.

Or you may be concerned about pregnancy or disease, and mutual masturbation is a way to achieve orgasm and closeness with another person without taking a risk. You might just want to try something different. Why not? It's your body. Have fun with it.

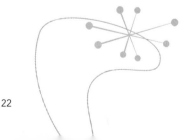

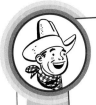

WELL, LOOK WHO FINALLY MADE THE *Rodeo*

To wrap this up, masturbation is touching yourself to achieve sexual pleasure. It's **FUN**, **FREE**, and **HARMLESS**, doesn't hurt anyone, and can help you sleep; if everyone masturbated (especially politicians), the world might just be a better place. So get to know yourself intimately. It will help you **RELAX**, you will learn what **TURNS YOU ON** and off, and it may even make you a **BETTER LOVER** when you have a partner or two in the room with you.

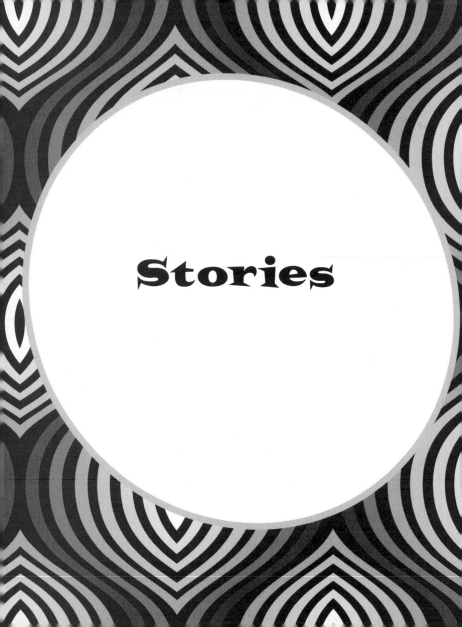

Stories

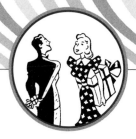

A New Toy

Anne Alexander

L ily could hardly wait to get home. She sat in the back of the cab, clutching her bag to her chest. She wanted to take it out and look at it, but she thought she better wait to get inside her apartment—or at least to the elevator.

Finally the taxi driver pulled up in front of her building. She gave him a handful of bills and rushed out of the cab and past the doorman. Once she was on her way up in the quiet elevator, she allowed herself to peek into the bag.

It hardly looked like a sex toy, really. It was almost demure there in its little purple box. She was glad the clerk had opened the box and put batteries in—she'd be able to just get right to it once she got inside. Lily knew Steve wouldn't be home. Not that she didn't want him to know about it or wouldn't show it to him later, but she thought her first time should be solo, away from her boyfriend's curious eyes.

She had it on good authority that this particular model was the best vibrator on the market. She'd asked Kara, her most sexually adventurous friend, about the best kind to use if she didn't actually want something penislike, just a vibrator. "The Love Bullet. No doubt about it," Kara had said without even pausing to think about it. So now, a week later, Lily had gone to the Pleasure Center, a bit embarrassed but mostly excited, and bought it.

Finally! Her floor! Her anticipation was rising with every passing minute. She unlocked her door and went inside.

Lily went immediately to the bedroom, taking off her coat and scarf on the way. Once inside, she shut the door and contemplated locking it. Nah, she thought. Steve won't be home for hours. She took the box out of the bag and then took the little gold vibrator out of the box. She turned it on and felt it buzz in her hand. "Weee!" she said aloud to no one. She turned it off again and set it down on her nightstand, then started taking off her clothes.

She pulled off her boots and socks, then unzipped her jeans, slid them over her hips, and kicked them off. She pulled her sweater over her head and threw it on a chair, then shook out her hair. Now down to her pink bra and panties, she pulled down the duvet and got into bed, pulling the blanket up only as far as her thighs. Lily figured she'd be warm enough soon.

She turned on some music—Prince seemed appropriate for the occasion—and thought about lighting some candles but decided that would be corny. Okay, I'm ready, she said to herself after briefly considering turning on some porn and dismissing it as unnecessary.

She turned it on and felt it buzz a little. She started moving it to the already wet spot between her legs but pulled it away and turned it off at the last moment. I need to start a little slower, Lily thought. I'll romance myself a little. Ha!

She ran her hands through her hair and down her chest to her nipples, which she tweaked lightly through the lace and silk of her bra. She sighed, imagining being taken from behind, doggie-style. Steve liked it that way; what he didn't know was how much she loved it, being ridden roughly as he reached around and fingered her, slamming into her again and again.

Sometimes he got so worked up that he smacked her ass. She really loved that. Thinking of it now, she felt a jolt from her nipples to her clitoris, and she thought she might be almost ready to fire up the Bullet.

"Mmmmm," Lily moaned, taking her hands from her nipples long enough to remove her bra. She licked her fingers and moved them back to her hard buds, her slippery saliva feeling fantastic on her skin. Prince was really getting into it too: ". . . little red Corvette . . . baby you're much too fast. . . ." She moaned again. "Mmmm. . . ."

She kept her left hand on her nipple as she reached down into her panties with her right and felt how warm and wet she was. She twirled her fingers in her pubic hair for a minute, then dipped lower into her vagina. She was so wet, so hot. "Ohhhh . . ." she murmured, swirling two fingers into herself.

Lily moved her fingers up and found her clitoris, which was hard and sensitive as she ran her finger around it. She thought of Steve doing her in the shower, from behind of course, the hot water coursing down on their naked skin. He would pull out almost all the way, then ram all the way in again until his balls smacked against her with each wet thrust.

"Oops," Lily said, opening her eyes. I almost forgot my new toy!

She picked it up and turned it on to the high setting, then moved it over to her wet nipple. Ooh, she thought, that's too much. She turned it down to medium and moved it down her firm belly to the top of her panties. With one more inch, she was inside the silky, damp material.

Lily licked her lips and, still twirling her fingers around her left nipple, moved the little vibrator down to her wet opening, dipping it inside herself briefly and getting it lubricated. That feels funny there, she thought, keeping the toy inside herself for a moment more until she could wait no longer.

She moved it up to her clit, circling it around the sensitive bud several times and thrilling at each tingly feeling of pleasure that ran through her whole body. "Mmmm," she purred again. She thought of being in the shower with Steve again, but this time she was on her knees in front of him, sucking his beautiful cock into her mouth again and again as he held the back of her head and moaned softly, smiling and about to come in her mouth.

"Oh, oh," she yelped, moving the Bullet faster over her clit and pulling on her nipple. She arched her back and spread her legs. She was sweating now as she strained toward her ultimate pleasure. In her mind, Steve was pounding into her as he moved his fingers on her clitoris, getting ready to come with her and fill her, but in reality, she moved the vibrator with lightning speed now, fast approaching her own climax.

"Yeah, yeah, babe, yeah," she whimpered, circling her nipple again. "Ohhh," she moaned as she stopped moving, held perfectly still, and came. Hard. She felt the miraculous feeling of letting go of all sense and tension, good feelings pouring all over her body as she held the vibrator still on her clitoris. She felt her orgasm ripple through her for a full minute as her insides contracted over and over again. "Ohhhh. Mmm," she sighed, spent and delighted.

Suddenly, she heard clapping. Her eyes flew open, and there was Steve, standing in the doorway applauding her with a massive erection straining the front of his pants.

She pulled the blanket up over herself. "When did you get home? How long have you been here?"

"Long enough, babe. Damn, I'm so glad I came home early. That was the hottest thing I've ever seen."

Lily blushed. "Well, I finally just went and got a vibrator, and I wanted to try it out. . . ."

"No need to make excuses. But do you have any energy left for me?"

Lily smiled. "Always."

VIDEO

J. M. Thompson

Terry stepped off the shuttle bus, walked around to the back, and grabbed his bag while handing the driver a tip. With his laptop bag over his shoulder, he grabbed the extended handle to his roller bag and headed through the automatic doors into the hotel lobby. Smiling at the desk clerk, he said in a quiet voice, "I have reservations for Anders, Terry Anders."

Within a few minutes, Terry had his room key card. The desk clerk said, "You'll be in room 1504. Just take the elevators at the back of the lobby." She pointed to the elevators while he grabbed his bag.

Terry got on the elevator. The doors quickly slid shut, and the elevator moved rapidly upward. When it reached his floor, the doors opened and Terry stepped into the hallway. He headed to the right and then slipped his key card into the door. The small light flashed green, and he pushed the door inward, dragging his rolling bag behind him. He moved the bag into the closet and stepped farther into the room, letting the door close behind him.

He eased the computer bag off his shoulder, unzipped it, pulled out his laptop, and placed it on the desk. He opened it, plugged the mouse cord into the USB port, and turned on the computer. Reaching back into the bag, he grabbed a flash drive and placed it next to the computer. As the computer started up, he kicked off his shoes, pulled off his shirt and pants, and sat down in the desk chair.

Remembering something, he spun in the chair, pulled a small set of earphones out of the computer bag, and plugged them in. Once they were plugged in and he saw the computer had finished its start-up ritual, he turned on the sound and plugged in the flash drive. When the window popped up, he clicked through several layers of folders until he found the exact file he wanted.

With a double click, he started the video file and then put the earphones in his ear, waiting for the video to begin. When it showed up in a small window, he clicked an arrow, and the window expanded to full screen, where he could see a slightly grainy view of a naked woman. She was in bed on her back, with her legs spread open.

Terry looked over the woman, her large breasts sagging a bit, her nipples jutting outward toward the viewer, her slightly rounded stomach rising and falling slowly as she breathed. Pausing the video, Terry smiled, admiring the familiar territory of his wife's body, remembering it as he had seen it last, a few days earlier. He clicked play and watched as his wife's hand moved down between her legs, her fingers parting her lips slightly, slipping inside and coating them in her wetness. As her fingers moved up to her slit again, opening it and finding her clit, Terry took his palms and began circling them over his nipples. With just a bit of movement, he could feel his nipples and cock harden.

His wife paused a moment, moving her fingers back and forth until they were comfortable on her clit, and then she began a slow circling movement. Terry watched intently as her hand continued to move, quickening the pace a bit. After a few moments he watched her move her hips just a little, lifting herself, pushing up to her fingers. As she continued, she began to move her hips a bit more, reminding him of how she moved when they made love as she lifted herself up to him.

A little later, Terry could hear a sound, a faint coo that soon was followed by a louder moan. He cock was hard now, but, teasing himself, he only touched his nipples, leaving his cock throbbing wantonly against his jockey shorts. His wife moaned again loudly and lifted her hips, moving her legs in and out. Yes, he could see and hear it now; she was coming and she whined loudly, quickly pulled her fingers from her clit, and closed her legs.

The video looped back to the beginning. As Terry slipped off his jockey shorts, freeing his cock, he could see his wife's fingers dip once again into herself and then move, glistening, up to her clit. Wrapping his fingers around his cock, he began moving his hand up and down the shaft as he intently watched his wife's fingers move over her clitoris. As she lifted her hips for the first time, Terry lifted his, remembering how turned on he had been when he filmed his wife doing this.

Terry savored the sensations that were building in his cock as he continued stroking, lifting his hips and thrusting forward whenever his wife lifted hers. As he listened to her first moan, he had to slow down his stroke a bit, wanting to time himself perfectly. His hand moved slowly now as he felt himself on the edge, hanging there, waiting for that special moment. Another moan and he stroked a bit faster; yes, the feeling was so good as it ran down his cock to his balls.

And then it happened. She began her whine, that incredibly beautiful sound she made when she came, when her body felt the intense pleasure shoot from her clit and take her completely. Terry's hand moved quickly, and he felt the hot splash hit his stomach once and then again. He continued stroking as he watched his wife pull her hand from her clit and close her legs, simply enjoying the sensations that filled her. Terry slowed his hand as his juice continued oozing down over his fist.

He grabbed a nearby towel and cleaned himself up as he watched the video loop once again and his wife's fingers slipped inside herself. The video continued playing as Terry sat back, catching his breath as his wife once again began lifting her hips. He left the video playing until she came again, then he clicked it off and got dressed for dinner. After dinner, he'd give her a call and perhaps tell her about the wonderful video he watched that afternoon.

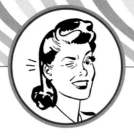

Heavy Breathing

Wolf Feather

My wife has always been much more of a heavy breather than a screamer or a moaner. While I quite enjoy the moans and especially the screams of a woman in the throes of ecstasy, the heavy breathing is also sexy in itself. The very few times my wife has screamed in pleasure all followed lengthy periods of heavy breathing during which I would arouse her to the brink of orgasm, then deny her the sexual release.

Fortunately, those were times when I had first secured her limbs to the bedposts, or else she definitely would have choked me to death for denying her again and again and again.

When I returned early from work to get a jump on the weekend, it was clear that my wife had not heard me pull the car into the driveway or enter our small house, because she was nowhere in sight, yet her car was in the driveway. As

I approached the bedroom, however, I was very pleasantly surprised to hear her heavy breathing—it was faint from my vantage point but definitely enough to begin a telltale lengthening process within my slacks.

As quietly as possible, I moved down the carpeted hallway. My wife's heavy breaths sounded full of need, as if her quest for release was just about to reach a long-anticipated climax. Finding the bedroom door open wide, I looked in to find her on her back, lying across the bed, her head hanging over the side, her face a bit red from the blood pooling in her head, the ends of her rust-colored hair brushing the carpet. I knew from both her comments and the reaction of her body just how much she enjoyed having sex with her head unsupported like this, as the pooling blood gave her a more "heady" sensation in the experience.

Her eyes were closed, but her mouth more than compensated. The breathy sounds escaping past those plump, red-painted lips were hard and short, almost staccato notes sounding in nearly perfect rhythm with the bucking of her naked body against the actions of her hands. Yet somehow, the earphones had not fallen from her head.

I followed the cord of the earphones to the small MP3 player beside her on the bed. Clearly, my wife could not hear me, so I stepped into the bedroom, not wanting to disturb her wonderful lewd display of carnal femininity yet curious about what had brought her to such a frenzy. Bending over the bed without touching it so that I would not alert her to my presence this early in the afternoon, I recognized the track title as one of our favorite sound files downloaded from a sex sounds website: a track of a woman being (supposedly) double-penetrated and perpetually screaming for the entire eight-plus minutes of the file as another woman's barely heard voice provided encouragement for her to keep screaming and for the two men to keep fucking her.

She plunged a thick dildo repeatedly into her dripping body as her other hand worked her clitoris furiously. As a multiorgasmic woman, my wife could conceivably ride the tidal waves of primal pleasure for some five minutes, which meant a great visual treat for me. I stepped back from the bed and leaned against the wall, gently caressing my erection through my slacks while I enjoyed the vision of self-lust.

Yet, although the sight before me was indeed grand, it was the heavy breathing that truly attracted my attention. Her breathing—and the rapid rise and fall of her firm breasts—was becoming more and more erratic, her exhalations sharper and slightly louder, yet she was still not quite at the point where her conscious mind would let go of her self-control and allow her beautiful siren voice to sing unabashedly (and unknowingly) to me.

Then it finally happened: her body stiff yet quivering visibly, the initial orgasm drowned her senses. All breathing ceased, and her heart probably stopped beating as well. Her eyes snapped open and she happened to be looking directly at my hand upon my crotch, but from the faraway, glassy look in those large hazel orbs, she clearly was unable to see anything through the haze of her all-consuming carnal release.

That image of my sultry wife instantly seared itself onto my brain, a vision never to be forgotten. The prominent nipples appeared to be as hard as the small rings piercing them. Her skin seemed to shine, and not just from the sweat that had formed upon her. The end of the long fluorescent green dildo appeared explicitly obscene in her hand. Her rusty hair seemed to form a curtain hiding the inappropriate treasures we stored underneath the bed.

Just as suddenly as she had stiffened, the beauty on the bed once again became a study in motion, pistoning the dildo inside her and furiously torturing her clitoris. Her heavy breathing—and certainly her heartbeat—again resumed, this time louder than before. Her eyes closed again, my wife bobbed her head up and down and shook from side to side, causing the rust-colored curtain to shimmy. The movements of her breasts were almost mesmerizing, enhanced by the small ring of silver attached to each proud, attention-demanding nipple.

I watched with rapt interest, devouring the lewd scene before me, inhaling the scent of excited femininity, and savoring the sound of her heavy breathing. Through the slacks, I stroked myself more urgently, such was the effect of the libidinous display before me.

The beautiful hazel orbs opened again, looking directly at my hand-covered crotch. The haze of sexuality had apparently lifted just enough for her to realize that she was no longer alone, and an exhalation that had begun as a soft grunt whiplashed into a startled scream, but then even that snapped into an orgasmic cry as she inflicted another climax upon her writhing body.

Since she knew that I was with her, I debated whether I should join her—perhaps take over control of the dildo, or pay loving attention to her chest, or just kneel beside the bed and stroke her reddened cheeks as I swallowed her screams.

I chose the latter, inhaling her hot excited cries as wave after wave of primal pleasure surged through every cell of her being.

When her hands at last fell limp upon the bed and the florescent green dildo slowly slid out of her thoroughly lubricated sex, I sat back on my heels. Knowing she was in no condition to move to a better position, I held her head so it was horizontal with the rest of her body, allowing for a more proper flow of blood. Slowly, the color drained from her face as I kissed her sweat-covered cheeks and forehead, my eyes riveted on the unsubtle rise and fall of her chest, my ears trained on her renewed heavy breathing.

My wife never asked why I had come home early or how much of her frenzied display I had seen. She did blush profusely as she dressed, and she kept looking at me with an embarrassed expression throughout the evening. The only mention of the lewd scene occurred that night in bed as I held her snugly to me:

"Did you enjoy the show?"

I never answered verbally, but even in the darkness, I believe she heard my smile.

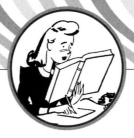

LIBRARIAN

J. M. Thompson

I guess it all started when they extended the hours for the library. To be honest, I'm not sure why they did it. I mean, it wasn't busy during the hours we originally were open. Perhaps they thought if we were open longer, people might be more apt to stop in at the new times. Well, it didn't work, and all that happened was that Ms. Harrington and I simply had to look busy while doing practically nothing.

Ms. Harrington was the librarian, a sometimes grumpy but normally somewhat pleasant middle-aged woman. Needless to say, as quiet as it was there, Ms. Harrington and I had the place looking better and running more efficiently than it ever had. The books were back on the stacks within fifteen minutes of being returned, new books usually were cataloged within an hour or two, and there wasn't a bit of dust anywhere.

Even after all the cleaning, stacking, and cataloging, there was still a lot of time when we were either waiting for someone to come in or waiting for one or two people to make their choices and check out. I usually spent those down times sitting at the checkout desk holding a book below the level of the upper counter so the customers couldn't see me reading. Ms. Harrington would see me reading, but as long as everything was stacked, cataloged, and nicely dusted, she wouldn't say anything about it.

Today, for some reason, she walked around behind the desk and said, "Reading again?"

Closing the book quickly, I said, "Ugh, yes, just until some customers come in."

"Relax. I mean you have all the books stacked . . ."

I nodded.

". . . and all the new ones are cataloged . . ."

I nodded again.

". . . and everything is dusted?"

"Yes, ma'am."

"Well, then, it's okay to read. It's just that, well, what is it you're reading?"

"Oh, just something I found in the new releases, a thriller."

"Jerry, don't you know there are some magnificent books in our stacks here that absolutely must be read, but everyone goes to the new releases as if everything else is outdated. That best seller may be popular, but what are you getting out of it but a few thrills?"

"The critics seemed to have liked it."

"Critics? Have you read the full critique or just the blurbs?"

"Just what's here on the book."

"That is advertising, complete spin. Why not look up the actual reviews and see what was said? You might end up with a different outlook."

"But what books are you talking about?"

"Here, I have a list I often pass out to people. These are some of the books we have that scream to be read, books that everyone should read in their lifetime. Look it over and see what you think," she replied, handing me the list and then walking back toward her office.

As I picked up the list, she paused and looked back at me and said, "And Jerry, one more thing."

"What's that?"

"Calling me Ms. Harrington is simply too stuffy. Just call me Denise, okay?"

"Okay, Ms. Har . . . uh, Denise."

She disappeared into her office as I unfolded her list. Looking down the list, I saw Hemingway, Steinbeck, Tolstoy, but also a number of books by Anaïs Nin, D. H. Lawrence, Henry Miller, Marguerite Duras, and even Georges Bataille. I moved my book aside and wandered out into the stacks.

Over the next few days, I started reading some of the books she had listed. Not sure I was ready to handle Hemingway or Tolstoy, I had grabbed Nin's *Delta of Venus*. After reading a little, I was surprised it was available here at the library. I mean, it was pretty hot. Anyway, I often found myself needing to make adjustments to my pants as I got an erection reading the passages.

I would look around, making sure no one was watching, and then, as nonchalantly as possible, reach down and adjust my cock.

It was after one of those adjustments that I thought I heard something, a slight cry or moan, and I was worried Ms. Harr—Denise might have hurt herself or something. I got up and walked back toward the door to her office and saw it was slightly ajar. Quietly, I opened it a bit more and was about to call her name when I saw her.

She was sitting on one of the cushioned chairs facing the one-way glass that looked out onto the checkout desk and book stacks. She was leaning back in the chair with her eyes closed, and I initially thought she was having a heart attack or something, but before I moved, I noticed she had one hand in her pants and was squeezing a breast with the other. I should have walked away, but I couldn't.

I couldn't see much other than the outline of her hand moving in her pants, but her hips were moving up and down and she continued squeezing her breast. She moaned and began moving her hand and her hips faster. Quite shocked at seeing a woman her age going so wild, I felt my cock bulging in my pants. Finally, she lifted her hips off the chair and arched her back, supporting herself with her shoulders on the back of the door as she came.

Her body quickly relaxed, and she settled back into the chair, breathing heavily. I immediately turned and headed straight to the men's rest room, slipped into a stall, closed the door, and pulled out my erect cock. Standing there in front of the toilet, I began stroking myself wildly while images of Denise playing with herself spun through my mind.

Almost immediately, I could feel the pleasure building inside me and moved my hand even faster. Looking down, I watched as the head of my cock appeared and then disappeared from my view. I came quickly and pointed my cock down at the toilet, watching it spurt once, twice, and a third time into the water. I dabbed up the rest with some toilet paper as it dribbled out of my cock.

I then headed back to the checkout desk and picked up my book. Several minutes later, I noticed Denise emerge from her office and head to the ladies' room. Her face seemed a bit flushed, and her hair was mussed up. After a few minutes, she came out of the rest room looking all prim and proper.

As she walked past me, she looked at the book I was reading and said, "Ah, I'm glad you took my advice on looking into the book stacks for something good. You know, you'd be amazed what you will find here in the library."

Looking up at her face and remembering how it had contorted in pleasure as she made herself come, I replied, "I know what you mean, Denise. I know what you mean."

Good Morning

Anne Alexander

I woke as I usually do, just before seven, when the alarm goes off. I lay under the duvet for a moment, dreading leaving the warmth of the bed for a cold winter morning of commuting and then work. I reached down and idly stroked my morning wood for a minute, and I thought of you, wishing you were here to stay in bed and play hooky with me.

After a few moments, I realized I better get moving or I'd be late, so I hopped out of bed and, without bothering with a robe, ran quickly to the bathroom. I turned on the shower and let it steam up in there a bit as I relieved myself and rubbed my eyes, then stepped into the warm spray.

Reaching down with the soap, I realized that my morning erection hadn't gone away after I peed and that I was still thinking of you . . . the way you stroked me, the way you kissed me, the way your eyes looked when you took my hard flesh into your mouth and brought me to the height of pleasure, sometimes in this very shower. Oh, how I missed you at that moment and how I wished you were still with me.

I washed the rest of my body, using the bar of soap to suds up my smooth chest and muscled arms, stopping to run a soapy finger around each nipple. Then I brought the soap to my ass, running it over each cheek and then into the crack. I felt myself open to my own finger, and I briefly became distracted and moved one digit inside, thrilling at how easily it slid in because of the lather. It feels so good that I moved it in and out a few times, thinking of you again and how much you loved to please me this way.

Snapping back into reality, I tried to get back on track and finish up as I moved my hands down each leg, working the soap through the wiry hair there. I moved my hands back up again to my crotch, where my erection just would not go away. I gave in and stroked myself for a brief instant but then began to rinse off.

As I picked up the shampoo, the alarm went off, and it was still set to that stupid soft rock station you hated. Of course this morning Air Supply was playing, making me think of that one year when you serenaded me so sweetly on my birthday: "All I need is the air that I breathe, and to love you. . . ."

What a cheesy song! But yeah, it made me think of you anyway, and I started to laugh as I washed my hair, rubbing my scalp and feeling all the tension leave my body. That is, all the tension except what was concentrated there between my legs.

"Oh, screw it," I said out loud. I could just walk a little faster to work—it was only fourteen blocks, after all, and I'd rushed to make it on time before. There was that time you'd surprised me with breakfast in bed and we hadn't eaten more than two bites before we were tasting each other. With syrup. Mmmm.

I rinsed my hair, then gave myself fully up to the memory of that morning. It wasn't even a year ago, and you'd just finished culinary school and had gotten a job at a great restaurant downtown—entry level, but a step in the right direction. You'd been cooking for me constantly, not that I was complaining, and you woke me up with fresh coffee and a plate of steaming challah French toast with real maple syrup and bacon. I wasn't sure I could've ever loved you more than I did at that moment, but then you kissed me. I was still mostly asleep, but I kissed you back; it was like second nature, and I didn't need to be fully cognizant to do it.

"Look at this," you said, pulling back the covers to reveal my morning wood, which was always in evidence in those days. Before I could respond, you'd put down the breakfast tray and begun playfully tugging my penis. Soon you got serious, though, and began a thorough hand job, until I stopped you.

Still in the shower, I stopped fighting the urge and was stroking myself hard, moving my hand in a tight fist up and down the shaft, using the water to keep it wet and slippery. Shit, that felt good.

I thought back to your questioning look as I moved your hand away from my cock that morning and pulled you down onto the bed with me, feeling your erection on my leg and wanting to feel it in my mouth. But I kissed you first, and our tongues danced a while with each other's lips and teeth. Soon you reached down and tugged off your own pajama bottoms, and we were both naked, the smell of breakfast and sex all around us. Speaking of breakfast, I picked up the syrup and poured a tiny bit on your belly. It was warm, and you jumped a little, but I held you down and licked the syrup out of your navel, savoring the taste of it and you together. And then I kissed down your belly and found your hard cock with my lips and engulfed you in my warm, sweet mouth.

I grunted in the shower, the hot spray and my hot body working together to get me off. As one hand furiously jerked my meat, the other reached behind me to my ass. I snaked one finger up there and nearly lost my balance it felt so great. "Oh yeah, oh yeah," I said out loud. This was going to be good.

You could never stand to be pleased and not do anything for me at the same time, so you sort of scooted around and took my cock in your hand as I sucked you. The feeling was so good. It was exquisite. I never wanted it to end. I felt the head of your cock hitting the roof of my mouth as I stroked your balls with my hands, wanting to taste your load on my tongue. I sucked faster as you started moving your hips, thrusting to meet me on the downstroke. I began thrusting too as you increased your stroke.

In the shower, I was barely holding on, wanting to have my release with us in the memory of that morning, so I slowed my stroke down a bit and stopped wiggling the finger in my ass. I took a breath.

But we were still going at it, and I looked up from your cock to see you swirling your finger around in the maple syrup. You tightened your grip on me with one hand as your other reached around my ass to my crack. All the while, I was licking the head of your dick as my fist moved up and down the shaft. When I felt your syrupy finger work its way into my ass, I couldn't hold out any longer, and I let go, shooting jet after jet of thick fluid onto your chest and belly. You smiled at me but then closed your eyes. The sight of my climax was too much for you; you couldn't hold out. You had to have your own. Even as the final spurts wracked my body, I closed my mouth over the head of your cock to catch your juice, swallowing every drop as you moaned and bucked. "I love you," you sighed.

"I love you!" I said in the shower, feverishly gripping my dick and coming into the bathtub. "I love you," I said again as the last few drops of my orgasm trickled out and were washed away by the cascade of water. I rinsed off and turned off the water, remembering how we ate the cold French toast and drank the lukewarm coffee, thoroughly satisfied.

I got dressed quickly for work then, thinking that wasn't such a bad way to start the day.

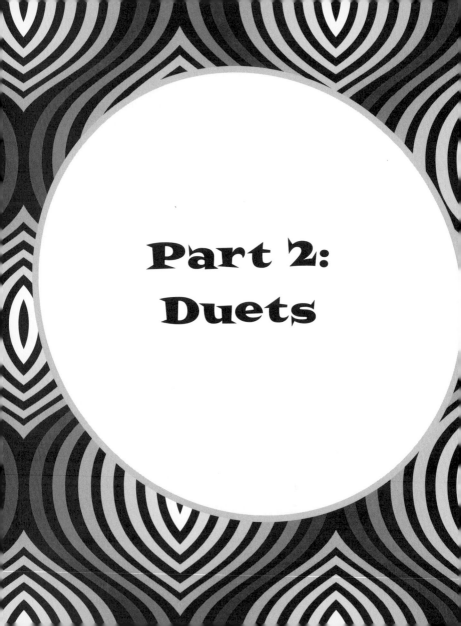

Part 2: Duets

Sex is best when it's one on one.

—*George Michael*

Most people like the idea of partnering with another person, at least for a little while. Some people like the idea of having sex with the same person for the rest of their lives—or as long as they're able to maneuver it. Maybe you're one of those, or maybe you'd rather play the field for as long as there is a field and you have play left in you. Either way, you will find yourself in bed (or on the floor, or on a table, or in an airplane rest room) with someone other than yourself, and it will behoove you to know what the heck to do with that person.

Lots of folks seem to think being with just one other person day in and day out has to be boring or routine or even sexless—and you may be one of them. We're here to tell you, though, that it's just not true. Sexuality offers a cornucopia of delights that only grows richer and more varied the more experience you have—and the more you explore your partner's body, turn-ons, desires, kinks, and pet peeves. But if you crave new, unexplored terrain and are not content to settle down for more than a month, a week, or heck, even a day with just one special someone, that's fine too, as long as you're safe and happy. There is certainly more to life than monogamy.

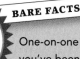

BARE FACTS

One-on-one sex can be fulfilling and exciting whether you've been with your partner for the last fifty years or just since the last subway stop.

There aren't any rules, and the only limits are your imagination and desires. Say sayonara to the standard missionary position and try doing it doggie-style in the shower or get a sex swing and string it up in the dining room. As long as your partner's into it, who's to say it's not okay? Not *The Big Bad Ass Book of Sex*, that's for certain.

COMMUNICATION

If you're openly communicating with your partner and playing it safe, there's no reason not to explore every facet of what our weird and wonderful bodies are capable of doing.

Whether you're new at the sex thing or ten thousand orgasms in, there's always more to learn about sharing sex with another person, and a refresher course never hurt anyone. Let's start with the basics, shall we?

LISTEN UP, THIS IS IMPORTANT

You might prefer to start your sexual encounters with intercourse and then get to the kissing and touching later on (or avoid that altogether), but we think a majority of humans like the buildup, so flirt, hold hands, giggle, talk, and then . . . kiss.

KISSING

Some people like kissing, and some people *love* kissing. Others barely tolerate it. Some say they can get off on kissing alone. No matter where you fall on the kissing continuum, you ought to know how to do it well enough that you don't asphyxiate or drown another person or yourself. It's not hard, but it does take a certain amount of finesse to get the breathing correct.

First of all, make sure the person you want to kiss wants to kiss you back. This might involve asking or following verbal and nonverbal clues.

DON'T BE A JERK

Unwanted kisses are never good kisses regardless of your technique.

Once you've got a person to kiss who'll kiss you back, start with light touches of your lips to his or hers. Kisses should be soft until the urgency grows and the pressure almost has to intensify. You'll feel this happen. You might like to open your mouth and let your tongue join in on the fun, but don't do this immediately. Like all things sexual and sensual, it's best to work up to more intense kissing. Don't plunge your tongue into your partner's mouth, either; start with feathery, almost tentative licks. If your partner is more conservative tonguewise, take your cues from him or her.

You may find it difficult at first to work out when to breathe during kissing, but try to breathe normally and you should do just fine. If you're really having a tough time, you can stop and start again in a few seconds or minutes. You can kiss a neck or earlobe in the meantime.

Speaking of necks and earlobes, those are great places to kiss. Cheeks, noses, and even eyelids are also popular, but generally it's a good idea to do it once, gauge the reaction you get, and do it again only if you receive positive feedback. Or, depending on how comfy you are talking about it, you could just ask. As with lips, these areas should be kissed lightly and with only a reasonable amount of saliva involved.

How much saliva is too much? Here's a good rule of thumb: you shouldn't need a towel at any point during the kissing process.

You might like to kiss other areas as well, such as collarbones, breasts, nipples, tummies, thighs, bottoms, genitals, legs, and feet. These are all great spots to kiss, and most folks like attention of varying degrees all over their bodies.

DON'T BE A JERK

You'd be hard-pressed to find a single person who likes a whole tongue shoved in his or her ear. It's just not preferred. Don't do it (unless someone asks specifically—and if that happens, please let us know; we've never heard of that as a preference).

As far as genital kissing goes, we're filing that under "oral sex," and it will be discussed a bit later in this part. For the other stuff, personal preference is really what it's all about. Once you're naked with another person, you should be able to talk to him or her about what parts of your body you like to have kissed and what parts you'd rather he or she avoid like the plague. Or you can show which ones you like and don't through reactions. (These can be verbal or not; examples include "Yes! Yes! Yes!" and yanking your elbow away as your girlfriend French kisses it for all she's worth.)

Speaking of nudity, that brings us to . . .

GETTING NAKED

Nudity with another person may really freak you out, or you may be an exhibitionist who loves to bare it all whenever possible—maybe you're one of those oddballs who like to prance around the locker room in the altogether, making more modest folks uncomfortably avert their eyes. Perhaps you are comfortable not wearing clothes only with your significant other or can be fully relaxed while naked only in utter darkness. No matter what your feelings on nudity are, there's no question that taking off all your clothing in the presence of another person and then fooling around with each other's bodies is an intimate and personal thing to do. It ought to be. Here are some things to remember when you do it.

Everyone is different. We're not saying everyone is beautiful, because that's just not true. But everyone is different, and the person who is about to see you buck-naked may not even notice things you don't like about your body. Just as the things you like about that person may be the things he or she hates the most. He may be uncircumcised and feel funny about it; she may have extra-large nipples and be embarrassed. But some women prefer uncut men, and some men think big nips are a huge turn-on. People are strange, and bodies are weird, imperfect things; we all have them, and we all have things we don't like about our own. Remember this and be sensitive. Lots of times, whoever you're with is thrilled just to see another person naked.

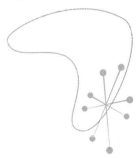

Unless there have been visits to a plastic surgeon, you and your partner are working with what Mother Nature gave you. There is no proof anywhere that the size of a penis or breasts negatively affects sexual pleasure from a physiological standpoint. Sure, some folks may like the look of big knockers or a long, thick dick, but lots of people with tiny breasts and small penises enjoy wonderful, satisfying sex lives.

Regardless of common sense, scientific facts, and all the anecdotal evidence you can stand, there still may be insecurity issues involving penis and breast size. That's normal. What's not normal or healthy is letting those insecurities keep you from enjoying being naked and sexual with other people. If any of these problems exist, talk about them together. If that's not enough, find a therapist to talk to. There is no reason to have unsatisfying sex, especially if it stems from feeling bad about your body, which can affect all kinds of aspects of your life. So sort it out and take it off!

EROGENOUS ZONES

We're not going to give you an anatomy lesson here; that's not why you're reading this book. There are tons of other books out there you can read if you want to know about seminal vesicles or Bartholin's glands. That said, though, there are some areas you should know about. Our bodies are rife with spots that love to be touched, that ache to be kissed. Some of these we can touch and maybe even kiss when we're alone, but some are made to be enjoyed by another. Here's brief rundown of our bodies' hotspots, broken down into primary (i.e., sex organs) and secondary (i.e., areas that just feel nice when paid attention to).

The Gräfenberg spot, or G-spot, wasn't named after the lucky soul who discovered its erotic potential—the seventeenth-century physician Regnier de Graaf—but after Ernst Gräfenberg, a mid-twentieth-century gynecologist who also reported this easily aroused zone.

Primary

* The *penis* is the main one for a man, obviously, and in general it doesn't need to be treated delicately. Most men touch themselves with a fair amount of pressure, but you can kiss and lick it gently or suck and stroke it roughly, and chances are, it won't complain as long as you keep paying attention to it. The *frenulum* is particularly sensitive; it's the area right under the head on the underside.

* The *clitoris* is at the top of a woman's vulva and is the only piece of human anatomy—male or female—that exists purely for pleasure. So use it! Women are pretty different when it comes to how hard or softly they can stand to be touched here, so start slowly.

* Some folks say women's orgasms originate in the *vagina*; some say they don't. We say, Who cares? If you like having yours touched and penetrated during sex, then go for it. The *G-spot* is just inside the vagina, at the top, and some women claim that orgasms originating here are the most intense.

* *Nipples* are sensitive for most women and for some men. Both may like theirs tugged or kissed, but it's best to try it out and see before you make it part of your sexual repertoire.

* Lots of men like their *testicles* played with, and lots play with them whenever they get the chance.

* The *labia majora and minora* (the outer and inner lips of the vulva) are sensitive areas for a lot of women.
* The *perineum* is the strip of skin between the scrotum and the anus, and lots of men and some women like to have theirs stroked. But proceed with caution, as it may be ticklish.
* Some people may like a finger or tongue in the *anus*, and some may not.

LISTEN UP, THIS IS IMPORTANT

Butt play is often considered taboo, so it might be good to approach the subject (or the ass) tentatively—at least until you've tested the waters and are sure the backdoor is open and ready for visitors.

Secondary

* The *mouth, lips,* and *tongue* are all very sensitive; see above on kissing.
* Most people, male and female, like to have the *neck* stroked and kissed—and even gently sucked—during foreplay and sex. Steer clear of sucking so hard that you break blood vessels and dark bruiselike marks appear, though: Unless they have a fetish or enjoy wearing turtlenecks even in the summer, most people aren't fans of hickeys.
* Both sexes seem to agree that little kisses and licks around the *ears* and *earlobes* are nice.
* The *shoulders* are a great area to stroke and kiss—some people find this to be one of the most erotic spots on their bodies and get pretty worked up when they're rubbed or kissed here.
* Women and men alike sometimes enjoy being kissed or licked in their *armpits*, but be cautious: tickling may ensue.

* Stroking or licking the *inner thighs* is a winning move when taking a break from the rigors of oral sex.

* Lots of folks enjoy having their *feet and toes* kissed, sucked, or rubbed. But for all those who love it, there are probably an equal number who can't stand it as a result of ticklishness. As with everything, a partner's personal preference should rule.

* Some may enjoy a kiss or lick on or around their *belly buttons*.

* Finally, perhaps the most important erogenous zone for men and women is . . . the *brain*. That's right; if the mind's not into it, it won't be any good. So use your head when you get naked with someone. You may lose your head at some point, but make sure your brain agrees with your genitals or you may end up getting screwed.

BARE FACTS

Pretty much everyone loves a massage, and rubbing the back of a person you'd like to have sex with is often a surefire way to get him or her relaxed and in the mood. It's also a great way to start off an evening of nakedness.

TOUCHING EACH OTHER

Men and women are different. Whoa! What a revelation, right? Yeah, but sometimes the differences are subtle, such as how much one or the other likes to drink beer or wine or read books about the Civil War, and sometimes the differences are huge, night-and-day disparities such as how hard one or the other likes to be touched in an intimate way.

Generally men are fairly rough with themselves, grasping their penises firmly and moving their hands up and down quickly, using strong pressure. In contrast, women usually can barely stand for their clitorises to be touched, and certainly not until they're very aroused. Some like stronger pressure as they get close to orgasm, and some like only the area around the clitoris to be touched and can't stand having the bud touched directly at all.

This is a general rule, but as always, when it comes to specifics, ask your partner how he or she likes to be touched or how he or she masturbates or follow nonverbal clues. If your partner is the same sex as you, you have a leg up, as it were. But you should still ask, since personal preference always varies.

IT'S GETTING HOT IN HERE

So far, things are progressing nicely. You're touching each other's naked bodies and planting some well-placed kisses. So what's going on with your body now that things are heating up? Read on.

For the Ladies

After a woman has been fooling around with someone for a while, she'll start to notice that some outward physical things about herself have changed in addition to the tingly good feelings she'll be having all over her body, in particular between her legs. As she starts to get aroused, a woman may notice shortness of breath, or the skin on her chest and face may start to get a little pink. That's called sex flush, and it's more common in women than in men, and it's cute! So don't worry, you don't have a rash. Her breasts may swell slightly, too.

SECRET TIP

If a sex flush doesn't go away soon after sex, you may indeed have a rash. Seek treatment if that's the case.

A woman will also notice her lady parts feeling kind of squishy the more turned on she gets. This extra vaginal lubrication is caused by blood pooling in that area and serves two purposes:

1. It helps increase the possibility of getting knocked up.
2. It increases the enjoyment of sex.

We're mostly concerned with that second one because that's what this book is about.

BARE FACTS

If you want information on the first point above, get yourself a different book. (Perhaps *The Big Bad Ass Book of Babies* is forthcoming.) If you don't want information on the first point, make sure you're using protection.

Slipperiness makes sex feel better and makes it easier for a penis or another something to be inserted into a vagina. The added wetness also makes thrusting feel good. Think about it: All that thrusting would make for lots of friction—the unpleasant kind—without some lubrication going on in there.

Level of arousal is not always innately tied to how wet a woman gets. The amount of natural lube a woman produces as she gets turned on varies from woman to woman as well as in a specific woman depending on the stage of her monthly cycle she is in. Generally speaking, the more the better, but sometimes there may not be enough. This could be for any number of reasons, including but not limited to these:

✳ She is going through menopause.
✳ She's tired, stressed out, or not in the mood.
✳ Her natural lube isn't flowing as a result of the time of the month.

LISTEN UP, THIS IS IMPORTANT

The important thing to note here is that the reason for lack of natural lube is not always and doesn't ever have to be "She doesn't like what I'm doing" or "I don't turn her on."

Regardless of the reason, if dryness is something that happens from time to time, use a synthetic lubricant. If it's something that happens all the time, ask your gynecologist what's going on. But for God's sake, don't ignore it and have sex dry. It won't feel nice, and what's more, it probably will hurt. It's just not worth it when there are simple solutions to the problem.

For the Gentlemen

As a man gets turned on, he'll have the same shortness of breath as his female counterpart. He may even experience sex flush, though it's less common in men. The main one we all know about, though, is that his penis will fill with blood and harden, all the better to penetrate an orifice.

These days, it's almost impossible to get away from talk of erectile dysfunction. Seriously, people talk about it *all the time*. Imagine if they talked about vaginal dryness as often; imagine the commercials and products and medications and then the commercial spoofs and endless snickering. Okay, perhaps this is one instance where male-centrism works in favor of women.

This is all just to say that a lot of people talk about men not being able to get it up, but not a lot talk about why that is. It could be for any one of many reasons, including but not limited to these:

* He is tired, stressed out, not in the mood, or preoccupied with something else.
* He is nervous or has performance anxiety.
* He had an orgasm within the last hour or couple of hours.
* His spine is injured.
* He has another type of injury.

Again, the important thing to note here is that the reason is probably not "I don't turn him on" or "He thinks my technique is amateurish."

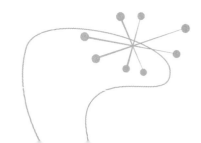

The occasional inability to get an erection is not the end of the world. It really does happen to most guys at one time or another, and it often has very little to do with the sexual situation they find themselves in at that moment. The one instance in which this may not be the case is when he's tense about pleasing another person and has performance anxiety, which can create a feedback loop of insecurity and inability to get hard.

Because ideas of manliness and the ability to please a woman are so often innately linked with erectile ability in men's—and yes, even women's—minds, the occasional flaccid penis really can do a number on a man's self-esteem and self-worth. But it doesn't have to if everyone remembers that a man can be manly even if he has a soft penis sometimes (because they all do at one time or another, and thank goodness; imagine all hard dicks all the time!). Or that it's possible for a man to please a woman and make her come even if his dick never makes an appearance. Or that often, if his penis stays soft, it has nothing to do with what she's doing or not doing. In short, it happens, it doesn't have to be made into a federal case, and you probably don't need to rush to your doctor demanding Viagra. Talk about it with your partner and move on.

However, if it happens all the time, that's impotence, and that is a sign of a more serious physiological or psychological problem. See a doctor if this is the case.

LET'S DO IT

You're physically and mentally ready—ready for the good stuff. Now you're confronted with a wonderful, varied, and perhaps slightly daunting array of fun things to do with yourself and another person's body. So many choices! How do you decide? Well, let's talk about them so you can make an informed decision.

In terms of all the things you can do that will make you feel good and make your partner feel good and will, generally speaking, lead to an orgasm for one or both of you, there are the following basic categories:

* Frottage, or dry humping
* Mutual masturbation
* Oral sex
* Vaginal sex
* Anal sex

Teenagers who are just learning about what feels good to them often practice *frottage*, and rubbing against another person does feel pretty good.

Mutual masturbation is touching yourself while your partner touches himself or herself—and you might touch each other, too—without having intercourse. It is often practiced by couples who are concerned about the risk of disease or pregnancy that accompanies penetrative sex.

Fellatio and cunnilingus are the two types of *oral sex*, and both involve mouth-to-genital contact. Folks think it feels good, and that's the main reason it's done, though some couples probably benefit from the fact that oral sex offers no risk of unwanted pregnancy.

When people talk about sex, they are most often talking about *vaginal intercourse,* in which a penis or penis-shaped implement is inserted in a vagina. It's a lot more fun than it sounds, trust us.

Anal intercourse has something of a bad reputation, but lots of folks like it. It's not just a man who enjoys the feeling of having his penis inside such a tight spot; women and men both seem to enjoy and even prefer having their backdoors done sometimes.

Frottage is fairly self-explanatory and *touching* has been pretty well covered already, so we're going right to oral, vaginal, and anal intercourse to discuss the ins and outs of it all.

ORAL SEX

Fellatio is using your mouth to lick, kiss, and suck a man's penis (and testicles, too, if you want). *Cunnilingus* is using your mouth to lick, kiss, and suck a woman's vulva, including the vagina, clitoris, and labia. It can be great fun for all involved, but it can be difficult to master, and not everyone is comfortable giving and/or receiving it. So say it with us: as with all things sexual, you must talk about it with your partner to make sure it is something both of you want. Once you know he or she wants it or wants to do it, you can figure out how you like it. That's the fun part.

DON'T BE A JERK

First and foremost, do not under any circumstances follow the oral sex guidelines adhered to for many years in porn movies. What looks hot on camera is *not* what feels good in reality, pretty much universally. Shoving your penis into someone's mouth over and over again so that he or she gags is generally not fun for the owner of said mouth (unless he or she asks for it in a role-playing or BDSM game; more on that later). Also, a woman does not generally prefer it when you stick your tongue out and shake your head wildly while grazing her clitoris. It may actually be uncomfortable for her, so be careful.

Helpful hints for giving a guy a blowjob:

* Start slowly with gentle licks and kisses around the base and head.
* Be firm when you really start sucking the shaft.
* Watch your teeth! Most men are enormously afraid of having their penises bitten during a blowjob.
* But then, some like to be grazed gently with the choppers, too.
* Stroke the shaft with your hands as you lick and suck the head. This will feel great, especially if he's well endowed and you can't or don't want to deep throat him. (Deep throating is not necessary, by the way. No one likes to gag, and he'll have a fine time even if you don't try to swallow his penis.)
* Don't forget his balls. A little tickle or kiss for the sac goes a long way.
* The frenulum, which is right under the head on the underside of the penis, is very sensitive. When he's close to orgasm, concentrate your efforts there.
* You don't have to swallow, but if you don't want to, make sure he'll let you know when you're about to have a mouthful.

Helpful hints for going down on a gal:

* Do not go straight for the clitoris unless she's already very aroused. Most women are extremely sensitive here, and some can't stand any direct pressure on the clitoris at all.
* Start slowly and build up.
* A woman may like a finger or two in her vagina while you kiss and lick around and on her clitoris.
* Try to keep your tongue soft; a rigid tongue may be uncomfortable or even hurt.
* Stubble may be irritating to a woman's most sensitive parts. Clean-shaven or a full beard is preferable.
* Alternate between licking around her vulva and concentrating on her clitoris until she's really close to orgasm.
* When she's close (she'll tell you, or you could stop a minute and ask), don't vary your movements too much. Keep it consistent until she comes.

Helpful hints for guys and gals who might like someone to pay them oral attention:

* You don't have to wax or shave your pubic hair, but keep it trimmed and neat. It's easier to concentrate on the good stuff if you're not spitting out hair.
* Keep clean. The reasons are obvious.
* If you are a woman who ejaculates when she comes, tell the person who is down there. Not all women do, so it may be a surprise and maybe not a pleasant one.

* Be vocal about what you like and don't like. Moans alone may not do it; you may have to say it out loud, in words. Come on, if a person is willing to put his or her face between your legs, you can use words to describe what you like.

COMMUNICATION

The main tip for anyone interested in oral sex is, say it with us: communication. Tell the person giving it what you like, and if you're giving it, tell the receiver what he or she can do to help you out.

Oral Sex Positions

There are lots of ways to go about fellatio and cunnilingus; it all depends on your preference (and how flexible you are).

* Lie on your back while your partner crouches, kneels, or lies between your legs and services you.
* Stand with your legs spread while your partner kneels before you and worships your private parts.
* Sit in a chair while your partner kneels at your feet and pays attention to you in a naughty way.
* Get down on all fours while your partner crouches behind you and loves you orally.
* A woman might "sit on" her partner's face as he eats her; that is, she can position her thighs around his head and give him great access to her pleasure center.

Lots of people like the good old 69 position for oral sex, in which both partners give and receive at the same time. This can be accomplished while both partners lie on their sides, or one can position himself or herself above his or her partner. (The latter works better in a man-woman scenario if the woman is on top; if she is on the bottom, it's difficult for him to maneuver his penis into her mouth, and pillows will definitely be required.) Sixty-nining is not for everyone, though; some folks feel that it's too much to concentrate on giving while they are receiving that kind of pleasure or that it's difficult to pull off physically. Try it if you like; if it's not for you, don't do it again.

BARE FACTS

Rimming is the slang term for oral-anal contact, or kissing and licking your partner's anus and crack. Some people like to do it, and some like to have it done to them. As with everything in the sexual realm, it's a matter of personal preference. If you want it and it's not happening, ask for it, and if suddenly your partner's got his or her tongue in your butt, don't be shocked if he or she wants tit for tat. Oh, and it goes without saying that rimming is a practice that demands good hygiene, so wash up if you want backdoor kissing.

VAGINAL INTERCOURSE

Usually when people talk about doing it, they're talking about penis-in-vagina sex. Obviously, there are tons of other things to do, and vaginal intercourse doesn't even have to involve a penis (for example, if it involves two women and some type of penis-shaped implement). But vaginal intercourse doesn't have to be—nor should it be expected to be—the main event in a sexual encounter (especially between, say, two men!). But just because it doesn't have to be the be-all, end-all of sex, that doesn't mean it's not deliciously fun and worthy of our attention in this book, so here we go.

Positions

There are literally hundreds of ways to set yourselves up to have vaginal intercourse. The only limits are your imagination and the physical shape you're in. The most variation you'll see has to do with leg placement, but here are some of the most popular sexual positions.

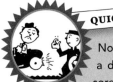

QUICK FIX

Not sure which position to try? Why not attempt one a day till you've found your favorite or you're too sore to keep trying?

* Basic missionary (man on top, woman's legs wrapped around him)
* Modified missionary (man on top, woman's legs straight up on his shoulders)
* Modified missionary #2 (man standing, woman lying on bed)
* Modified missionary #3 (man on top, woman's legs pushed back so her knees are near her ears)

* Modified missionary #4 (man on top but perpendicular to woman instead of parallel)
* Rear entry (she's on all fours, he's on his knees behind)
* Rear entry #2 (both on knees)
* Rear entry #3 (she's on his lap)
* Rear entry #4 (both lying on sides, like spoons)
* Rear entry #5 (she's on all fours, he stands behind)
* Woman on top (facing his face)
* Woman on top #2 (facing his feet)
* Woman on top #3 (both sitting up, facing each other)
* No one on top (partners lie with their heads away from each other and legs and genitals entwined)
* No one on top #2 (partners lie on their sides, facing each other, legs entwined)
* Standing up (woman wraps legs around man, man holds her up or props her against a wall)

LISTEN UP, THIS IS IMPORTANT

This may go without saying, but if you or your partner is in pain, seriously consider revising your plans. The fact that you read about a new position in a magazine or online doesn't mean it's for you.

You can vary any of these positions easily by substituting a bed for a chair, say, or using pillows below your head or booty. You might like to hang your head off the bed or sofa so you get a little light-headed, or you might rig up a sex swing in the bedroom and fuck in free fall. Or you might be into a little bit of discomfort during sex and try doing it on your hardwood floors or staircase. Any of these is worth trying, but if at any point one of you isn't having fun, stop and reposition. There's no reason to keep going if you don't like what's happening.

ANAL INTERCOURSE

Anal sex used to be considered a homosexual practice, nothing more. These days it seems that a fair amount of women and men enjoy having some type of phallus up their bums, and they seem to like it not just because it's thought to be taboo or naughty but because they like the feelings it produces. (Incidentally, studies and surveys have shown that gay men are more into fellatio than anal sex as a method of lovemaking.) But as long as both partners want to do it and everyone plays it safe, there's no reason not to enjoy anal intercourse if you care to. But it's not for everyone, and it doesn't have to be.

Slow and Steady

Anal intercourse takes a lot more prep work than the other kinds because anatomically, the anus was made to expel things, not take things in. Thus, you have to use lots of lube and lots of patience to get ready to fit a penis or phallus-shaped toy in there. You have to train the muscles to do something they're not used to doing, and that will take some time. Go slow and work up to it. You'll also want to withdraw anything you've put in your anus very slowly lest you pull out more than you put in. If you enjoy it, it'll be worth it, and if you don't, you don't ever have to do it again.

As opposed to the anus, the vagina was made to both expel and take things in. In fact, the vag is very tough and sturdy and it stretches and gets wet, whereas the anus is delicate, stretches less, and is not self-lubricating.

Safety is also something to consider more thoughtfully if you're planning to open up the backdoor. Everyone who does it should use a condom, and not just because of STDs (sexually transmitted diseases). Condoms will keep both partners clean in areas where cleanliness matters. So put a rubber on before you do it. Also, if you use a dildo up there, sheathe that, too, especially if it's one you also use vaginally. You don't want what's in your anus to be inside your vagina. Along the same lines, don't move your penis or dildo back and forth between holes. It's not a good idea hygienewise, because it can lead to bacterial infections.

Strike a Pose

The positions for anal intercourse are not terribly different from those for the vaginal variety, but you may need to do some shifting to make some of them work. These are the main ways to do it, but the variations are endless:

* Doggy-style is perhaps most commonly considered an anal sex position, and it certainly lends itself to that type of loving.
* The traditional missionary position works, but use some pillows under the rear of the receiver so that the giver can hit the target.
* The reverse cowgirl is great, too; that's when the giver is lying down and the receiver sits on top, facing away.
* Both partners might lie on their sides in spoon position, and the receiver can raise his or her top leg to accommodate the giver.

Lube!

As was mentioned above, the anus does not lubricate itself the way a vagina does, and so you'll need to use the synthetic kind. Don't go thinking you'll just use some of what's already produced in your vagina—it won't be enough even if you produce tons every time you're aroused.

So what to use? Water-based lubes are best. Oil-based ones can leave a coating inside your body that causes infections and breaks down the latex in condoms, rendering them ineffective, so don't use them. Silicone-based lubricants are newer and very popular because they're safe to use with condoms and seem to stay slippery longer, making them much better for anal sex. The only drawback? Some folks say they irritate their skin and are tough to wash off. Try a place a bit less sensitive than your vagina or anus (say, your arm or foot) and see how you react.

Whew. So that was the basics of one-on-one sex. Now that we've covered all that stuff, let's move on to commonly asked questions and issues a person might have when he or she is having sex with another person as well as descriptions of kinkier practices you might get into and ways to spice things up if you feel you might be in a rut. Onward!

ALL ABOUT ORGASMS

Reports and theories vary like crazy, so there's no definitive answer to where women's orgasms come from. Freud thought clitoral orgasms weren't as good as vaginal ones; Masters and Johnson talked about uterine orgasms; and G-spot orgasms seem to be all the rage these days, if vibrator sales are any indication.

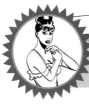
Men's orgasms are often taken for granted as something that happens as easily as a sneeze, but that's not really true. Some men take longer than others, some men hold back their orgasms on purpose, and some have a hard time coming at all. About the only thing that's consistent for men, though—in contrast to women—is that their orgasms all come from generally the same place and the same basic actions.

With all due respect to those who want to qualify and quantify orgasms, it doesn't matter where they come from, and it may not matter to you if you have one every time. How important they are to you, how often you want them, and how you get them is up to you and your partner, but lots of folks enjoy sex *even when they don't come*. That may be difficult for their partners to understand, especially if they're male partners, because generally they climax every single time and for the most part it's not terribly difficult for them. Sometimes, though, making a woman come requires more work. This is fine, except when your bedroom begins to resemble a scientific laboratory or Olympic training course and no one's having any fun.

Vaginal intercourse is super fun, and lots and lots of women really dig it even though lots and lots of women don't have orgasms from it. Or at least not it alone.

Many women enjoy oral sex very much but can't achieve orgasm that way. That's no excuse not to do it if you both enjoy it. This is true of all things sexual; if it's enjoyable, do it. If it doesn't lead directly to orgasm, so what? Orgasms are really, really great. No one's disputing that. But so are lots of other things about sex. So enjoy them all without putting so much focus on making somebody come that you forget to have fun.

This is not to suggest that it takes years of study and hours of practice to make every woman come or that every man will climax as easily as taking a leak. Some women come quickly, and some have multiple orgasms, which is a neat trick. Some don't, or won't every time, or may come after a few minutes of heavy petting one day and not even after a half hour of cunnilingus the next. Some guys may take a long time or sometimes not come at all. Some may not be able to come from a blowjob. Everyone's different, and each person may vary depending on the day or a mood or any of a laundry list of reasons. If your partner doesn't have an orgasm and he or she is upset, talk about it. If he or she is okay with not coming, don't worry about it. But talk about orgasms and their importance in your sex life, and be honest.

COMMUNICATION

Faking it is not a good idea. Most women have faked it in their sexual lives at one point or another, and that's no sin, but it's not a good habit to get into. If you're faking it all the time, you're not having much fun during sex, and you're also lying. If your partner feels good only after he's made you come and you're unable to come and you're faking it, there are a lot of things going wrong in your bedroom. But most of those things can be fixed with an honest conversation or several.

The Refractory Period

There is a stretch of time after a man has an orgasm during which he can't have another one, and it's called the *refractory period*. No one knows exactly why it exists, but it's probably neurological and it lasts anywhere from a few minutes to several hours. Women don't have a refractory period, though they may be too sensitive for further touching directly after experiencing a climax. So if your man can't get it up again immediately, it's not you, it's nature.

PERIOD PIECE

News flash: until they reach menopause, women menstruate approximately once a month for three to seven days or so. This means a sexually active woman has one of two choices:

1. She can abstain from vaginal intercourse during her period.
2. She can have vaginal intercourse during her period.

Both options are completely valid, and the choice can change from month to month—and certainly from woman to woman. How a woman feels about sex during her period is intensely personal and is based on any number of reasons and experiences, not least of which may be how a past partner or folks in general view sex during menstruation. Be sensitive, boys. It's a natural thing, and sure, it's messy, but there have probably been tons of times you were incredibly thankful a woman you were sleeping with got her period, so deal with it.

If you decide vaginal intercourse is just fine during her period, more power to you. Lots of women like it, and she'll definitely be slippery, so go for it. It's up to you and your partner, as always.

SAFETY

At this point in your life, you've probably had sex at least with yourself. You've probably also heard ad nauseam about safe sex, or safer sex, or protected sex, and you know what you need to protect your fragile body from when it comes to sex: AIDS, other sexually transmitted infections, and unwanted pregnancy. You've bought this book, and that's clearly a step on the way to protecting yourself from bad sex, so you should definitely protect yourself against the undesirable things that can come from unprotected sex. Here is a brief rundown of safer sex tools and practices that can ensure that you'll be doing it for a good long while.

✳ **NONPENETRATIVE SEX:** Mutual masturbation and frottage, as was discussed earlier, are both options, and as long as you're careful and no fluids are exchanged (which can be *very* difficult to ensure), this will prevent pregnancy and disease.

* **CONDOMS:** Condoms are made of latex or polyurethane, go on the penis during intercourse, and are very effective in preventing pregnancy and disease with no hormonal side effects. The only drawback is that some guys and gals say they can't feel the sensations as much. We say: you can't feel any sensations at all when you're dead. There are also female condoms, which are placed inside the vagina before sex. They work the same way as the male ones.

* **DENTAL DAMS:** These sheets of latex can be placed over the vulva during oral sex and prevent transmission of mouth-to-genital infections.

* **SPERMICIDE:** This is a jelly that kills sperm, and it'll help you not get pregnant but won't do much in the way of preventing disease, though some folks used to think it could. It's great to use in conjunction with condoms, though.

* **BIRTH CONTROL PILL, DIAPHRAGM, IUD, NORPLANT, DEPO-PROVERA, SPONGE, NUVARING, PATCH:** all these things will keep you from having a baby pretty effectively if you use them correctly. They will not, however, do a damn thing to keep you healthy and disease-free. If you are using any of these things and are not in a monogamous relationship, use a condom, too.

* **ABSTINENCE:** This means not doing it. But seriously? You bought this book. You're gonna do it. Just play it safe, okay?

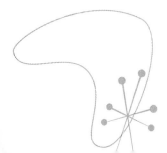

LISTEN UP, THIS IS IMPORTANT

Withdrawing the penis before ejaculation in hopes of preventing pregnancy or disease simply doesn't work. "Pulling out" means you've been in, unprotected, and it's not smart. Preejaculate has a less-concentrated amount of bad germs in it than ejaculate, sure, but the bad germs are still there. Oh, and perhaps so are the sperm, so you might get knocked up, too.

APHRODISIACS

Are there really foods and chemicals that affect sexual arousal? Maybe. Who knows? Whether it's science or the power of suggestion, there are some things that are said to enhance erotic pleasure, so what the heck. You might as well try these out and see how they affect you:

* Oysters
* Chocolate
* Wine
* Ginseng

* Spanish fly (cantharides)
* Kelp
* Arugula
* Green M&Ms

YOU'RE WELCOME FOR THE TIP

There are several drugs that may offer aphrodisiac effects, such as cocaine, ecstasy, LSD, and marijuana, but why risk the bad side effects or jail? Don't bother with them. Also stay away from opiates such as heroine and morphine, because they are anaphrodisiacs, which means they suppress sexual desire. Who wants that?

THERE'S MORE TO LIFE THAN VANILLA

Once you've mastered the basics, you're ready to move on to some wilder stuff, right? Something a little kinky, a little naughty, and definitely exciting! Here are some introductions to get you started.

SECRET TIP

If it intrigues you, your partner's into it, and you're taking safety precautions, there's no reason not to indulge in more risqué bedroom activities.

Toys

Who says sex toys are just for solo sexy times? If it's fun for one, why not incorporate a vibrator into one-to-one sex? Some men like to feel buzzing around their balls during intercourse, and if you can have clitoral stimulation during vaginal sex, why not?

A harness might be used with a dildo to create a strap-on, which allows a woman to be the giver in any type of intercourse. She might use it to have sex with another woman or to have anal sex with a man. Lots of men and women enjoy a feeling of fullness in their anuses during sex, and another toy that works for that is the butt plug.

This brings us gracefully to . . .

Anal Play

If you like a little backdoor attention but don't necessarily think you need something as big as a penis or a dildo in there, you might try rimming, which is literally kissing ass, or using fingers or smaller toys, such as butt plugs, for anal play. Some folks like something as big as a fist (hence "fisting") in there, and some can't stand more than a pinkie. Whatever the implement, it needs to be coated in lots of water- or silicone-based lubricant, and the watchword for anal play should always be "slow."

Many people believe that because of the prostate gland's proximity to the rectum, men enjoy anal play more than women. This may or may not be true, but it certainly doesn't mean all men enjoy it when you stick a finger up their bums. Some don't like how it feels, and some may worry that enjoying it makes them gay. Either way, if they don't like it, don't do it. The same goes for women, lots of whom report enjoying attention at their backdoors. But experimenting with the anal arena can't hurt (if you take it slowly).

SECRETS TO MAKE YOU LOOK GOOD

It can be awfully erotic to look at yourselves as you make love. But you needn't check in to a creepy sex palace to get the same effect; you can just get a full-size mirror and prop it up by your bed. In fact, doing it in front of a mirror might prompt you to try different things, which could be hot. Seeing yourself having sex might also prompt you to visit the gym more often, but that's another story.

Make a Movie

Tons of folks seem to love to watch themselves having sex. Imagine watching it when you can devote yourself to it, when you aren't busy doing something else, like actually having sex. Well, you can. All you need is a video camera or smartphone.

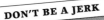

Once everyone's on board, set up the tripod, press record, and get down to business. Knowing you're being recorded could make that sex session one of the hottest you've ever had, so enjoy it! Then take a gander at your handiwork and see what you think. If it's hot, great. If it's not, delete it.

Role Playing

Perhaps you've always fantasized about being the galley slave to his pirate ship captain or the shy patient to her naughty nurse. There's nothing wrong with a little role playing—in fact, if it gets you off, there may be a lot right with it! Some folks find it lets them shed inhibitions; pretending to be someone else can really shake off those preconceived notions of what's good and what's not or how you *should* and *shouldn't* behave in bed.

Start simple: try being the teacher to your partner's misbehaving schoolboy or schoolgirl if that floats your boat. You needn't weave an intricate plot on your first foray; a few stern glances, a ruler, and an innocent shrug can get you pretty far with this one. Or start with something different that you've always wanted to try. It doesn't matter as long as you keep it simple to start with. You can graduate to more complicated scenarios once you're more seasoned and have figured out what you like. In fact, you might even incorporate dressing up in your role playing.

Dressing Up

Take the student-teacher role-playing game from above and build on it, maybe with knee socks and a plaid skirt, and you've got a grown-up game of dress-up. You can be as involved as you like with this. A few accessories will do the trick, but if you want to go the whole nine yards, go ahead. There are a few different kinds of dress-up games. You can dress up for a role-playing game, or you can just dress up because you want to, and these options are worth discussing.

First, you can dress sexy for your partner. Women might go with the old standbys of silky, slinky undies: bras, panties, garters, stockings, teddies—you name it—all accented with spike heels and vampy makeup. Men might get fancy undies, too, though they are slightly more limited in their choices. Some people really get off on this kind of dressing up, and some think it's a waste of time and effort because naked is just fine. But if you and your partner get turned on by it, why not?

SECRET TIP

One way to dress up is by putting on clothing not generally associated with your gender. Men might wear lacy panties or a dress, or women might put on a suit and tie. This type of cross-dressing doesn't mean you want to *be* the opposite sex; it might just turn you on to dress like this for a little while. It can certainly become a fetish, like anything, but here it's just a way to play with gender and get off.

Light BDSM

BDSM stands for "bondage, discipline, sadism, and masochism," and it has numerous devotees. It involves punishment, dominance, submission, and role playing in ways that often buck gender stereotypes and require leather outfits. Sound scary? It's not. At least the "light" variety you want to start with isn't. Like everything, it can get more involved and grow into a lifestyle or fetish, but in this section, we're just talking about a little spanking, a little dress-up, maybe some handcuffs, and a new outfit. See? Not so scary.

BARE FACTS

Most sexually adventurous people have at one time or another experienced a little light bondage, being blindfolded, dominance games, or playful spanking in bed. That's all light BDSM, and it's all just fine.

If you've never done any of this and you want to try it out, you don't need to spend hundreds of dollars at the local sex shop or spend a lot of time researching methods of dominance (unless you really want to). Try this: Next time you're in bed with your partner, tie his hands together with a silky scarf and go down on him. Then, while you're going at it doggy-style later on, tell him to spank you lightly. If you're into it, it should come naturally to you. If you're not, don't bother.

If you like that, though, you might work up to outfits and rules and collars and all that. You might want to dress him in a French maid's outfit and have him service you all day long while you occasionally whip his booty and tease him but never let him have an orgasm. He might want that, too, but you should definitely discuss it before you come home with an apron, a cat-o'-nine-tails, and a ball gag.

QUICK FIX

Most folks who practice BDSM have a "safeword" that one of the participants can use if he or she is uncomfortable with something that's going on. This is done because you might get carried away in character and leave your partner behind. Agree on the word ahead of time and make sure it isn't one that could lead to further confusion, such as "more," "yummy," or "don't stop."

If BDSM is something you and your partner really enjoy, there are all kinds of parties and clubs and societies you can go to or join. But start slow, with a scarf, maybe, or hot wax drippings, before you sign up for anything. (If your appetite for BDSM is not sated, flip to Part 5 for a more in-depth discussion.)

Finally, if you're feeling really adventurous, move on to Parts 3, 4, and 5 of this book for some *very* kinky ideas—including swinging and swapping!

REIGNITING THE PASSION

So you've been together for a while—maybe a few years, maybe forty—and you're looking to spice things up in the bedroom. There's no shame in that; in fact, it's admirable. You may have an orgasm every time, but that doesn't mean it's still exciting, and sometimes you have to work at that. Here are ten tips and tricks to rewhet your appetite for each other:

1. Buy a book of erotic stories. Oh, wait. You happen to have one in your hands! That's lucky. Turn a few pages and read a story. If you're feeling bold, read it aloud to your partner and see what develops.

2. Watch a porno movie or a regular movie with a few racy scenes in it if you're not ready for porn. Select one together and make sure it'll have something to titillate both of you.

3. Switch it up. Long-term couples can find themselves in a rut pretty easily. Do you always do it on Saturday nights? Try Sunday morning or Tuesday after work. Always in the bedroom? Try the shower or the living-room floor.

4. Take sexy photos. You can do this two different ways: one can take photos of the other, and vice versa, and you can share the entire experience together, which will be exciting and fun. Or one of you can set the timer and take photos solo, then present them to his or her partner as a sexy surprise. Either way, everyone wins.

5. Head outside. Whether it's camping in the mountains or a blanket in your backyard, al fresco sex is fun and exciting. A caveat: indecent exposure in public is illegal; be cautious and abide by the law.

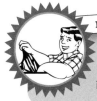

LISTEN UP, THIS IS IMPORTANT

Bug bites and/or sunburn can be murder on the more sensitive body parts. Use some lotion before getting into motion. Get some spray before having your way.

6. Buy a magazine with purportedly true tales of sexual adventure, such as *Penthouse Letters*, and read a story or two. It doesn't matter that it's probably all fiction; it might spark some creative bedroom play.

7. Go on a date. Dress up, go to dinner, go to the movies or a bar. Flirt with each other outside the house and talk about what you'd love to do when you get home. Then go home and do it!

8. Add some snacks. All kinds of fruit and dessert items can sweeten your lovemaking. Whipped cream and strawberries licked off each other might be nice, or if you don't have a sweet tooth, try champagne.

9. Have vacation sex—even if you're at home. Get a memento from the last time you were on vacation. It could be a song or a photo or something you wore. Talk about what it was like while you were away and get yourselves in that mindset. You may need to turn up the thermostat, but if you get into it, you should be able to turn up the heat, too.

10. When your partner arrives home, even if she's been gone only a couple of hours, greet her at the door completely naked. She'll know what to do with you—and it'll be naughty and fun.

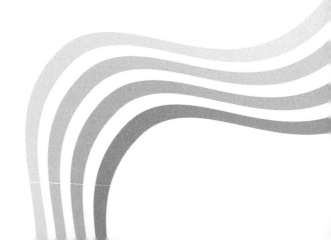

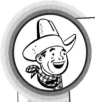

One-on-one sex does not have to be dreary or boring or the same every time. There are so many **DIFFERENT THINGS** you can do together and so many ways to **GET IT ON** and get off that really, there's no excuse if sex for you is dreary and boring.

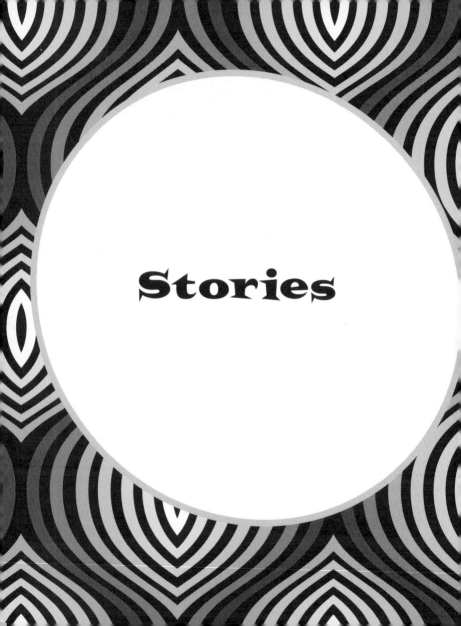

Stories

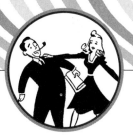

A Kiss

Tom Sullivan

Lu works down the hall from me, and I started fantasizing about her about five minutes after she joined our agency a few months ago.

The sleeveless blouses and tailored slacks she wore to work were just the start of her appeal. Her breasts looked full and heavy, and no other mother of three—including my wife—ever had a tighter-looking ass. She had a tiny, barely noticeable scar at the corner of her lip that made her mouth look like it was begging to be kissed. She wore her dark hair pulled back in a ponytail, and sometimes a stray lock would fall across her forehead and it was all you could do not to reach up and brush it back for her.

Lu had to cross my door to get to Cheryl's office; Cheryl was her team leader on a crucial pitch we were about to make.

After a while, I think she noticed that I always got up immediately, stood in my doorway, and watched that lovely behind of hers as she moved briskly down the hall.

In any event, even if she didn't consciously notice, I began to realize that she made a point of pausing to speak to the intern just outside my door whenever she walked by.

Alerted to Lu's presence, I'd station myself just inside my doorway to catch a glimpse. More and more often, she'd look up and give me the tiniest of smiles before breezing along on her way.

Was I imagining things, or did she seem to move a little more languorously and sensually these days? Was there a little extra sway in those hips meant for me?

This went on for several weeks until one fateful office happy hour. It's amazing how a couple of drinks can loosen someone up and make him a little forgetful about certain obligations.

Between us, Lu and I had eighteen years of marriage under our belts. Well, twenty-three if you counted my first one, along with the five years I'd had this go-round. I also had two stepchildren and a three-year-old daughter to complete the package. Lu was working on a lucky thirteen years with an English professor from the local university, and pictures of her three girls adorned the wall behind her desk.

Even so, with the subtle attention we'd been giving each other already, it was a short trip to outright flirting when bourbon fever kicked in.

Of course, the chances of spontaneous erotic combustion aren't real high on a Tuesday night when there are kids and homework waiting at home.

The next morning, though, the flirting continued, and over the last few weeks it's proceeded from there. From glances full of active curiosity to standing a bit too close in the elevator to letting our arms very, very carefully brush together while looking over a marketing plan draft, there's been a slow burn that's enjoyable just for its own sake.

At the same time, our conversation has gone from polite hellos to leaning into each other's offices for a few minutes of casual conversation.

When it was clear that neither of us was likely to file a sexual harassment suit against the other, a few double entendres found their way into our interactions.

Two weeks ago, things escalated a little more.

I'm notorious for my potty mouth. Other work settings are different, I know, but in the loose, creative atmosphere of an advertising agency, you can get away with a lot, and I admit to being downright vulgar at times.

Several of my coworkers credit me with the invention of the term "fucking fucker," but I'm pretty sure I actually heard it somewhere else first. That notwithstanding, I don't hesitate to let a "Jesus-fucking-Christ, that's the stupidest motherfucking-asshole-dumbass-motherfucker I've ever met" fly if the occasion warrants it.

To my delight, I found out that Lu was something of an artist in profanity herself. A tirade like the aforementioned one had exploded in a conference room full of equally irate copywriters, art directors, and producers when our latest pitch to a floundering client had been shot down. It continued with just

Lu and me in my office as we went back to the brainstorming board. Since we were both still cussing up a storm, Lu closed the door behind us and flopped down in my guest chair.

"Lu, I gotta tell you, that kind of talk is frankly quite shocking," I said in mock indignation.

"Stuff it, fucker; I know it turns you on," she retorted. We both broke out in giggles worthy of my thirteen-year-old stepdaughter and her friends.

"Turned on? I'm turned on, she says, and meanwhile I see her nipples poking through her shirt like a couple of walnuts," I said with a snicker.

"You don't want to go bringing up nuts of any sort, buster, with that bulge staring me in the face," she snorted, pointing at the very visible hard-on that was, in fact, at her eye level as I leaned back against my desk.

We kept this up playfully for a few more minutes before actually getting back to work, but from that moment on, dirty talk between us—in private, via text message, on the phone, even late at night at home through instant messaging—was not only tolerated, it was encouraged and one-upped and then pushed some more.

All that being said, Lu's been rather adamant that flirting, talking dirty, and sharing fantasies is as far as this is going. That's fine by me—one divorce is enough to last me a lifetime. More than anything, we both admit, our little oral affair has added fuel to pretty damn fiery sex lives at home.

Most guys don't even count it as officially getting laid until you've told your buddy about it, and the fact that my buddy was now a gorgeous thirty-six-year-old wife and mother with a body like a coed, an intellect like a physics professor, and a mouth like a sailor was just icing on the cake. I told Lu about how good my wife looked when she sucked my cock in the shower the other morning; she told me about riding her husband's face and licking her own juices off his chin and forehead. She picked out lingerie for my wife at Victoria's Secret online and dictated more and more of the outrageous text messages she was sending to her husband while he worked.

With that in mind, I picked up the phone just after lunch this afternoon and dialed Lu's extension.

"What now?" she answered huffily, and then chuckled. "What's going through that dirty mind of yours, bad boy?"

"Not nearly what I wish was going through my pants— namely, your hands," I said.

"That's a stretch even for you, darling. We're going to have work on your spontaneous sexy replies," she said.

"Maybe so," I replied. "But the reason I really called is to find out what your plans are to shock He-Who-Shall-Not-Be-Named later."

"Lingerie."

"Something new?" I asked, perking up.

"Something he hasn't seen yet," said Lu.

"And, much to my chagrin, neither have I," I sighed.

This got another chuckle.

"And you won't anytime soon," said my partner in witty repartee.

"Soon? That implies that at some point your panties will be mine!"

"Dream on, lover," she replied.

"So just what are you going to do with this lingerie for the lucky boy?"

"Before he leaves for his conference tomorrow, I'm going to put my sexiest panties in his briefcase. . ."

This elicited the usual intelligent reply from me: "Mmmmm."

". . . and when he lands in Denver, his little BlackBerry will chirp right away with the message that says I'm not going to wear any until he gets back next week—but that I packed a few dirty ones in his suitcase for him to stroke his cock with."

"I like it, Lu."

"Knew you would, bad boy, just like my husband will," Lu said, and I could hear the smile in her voice. "I especially like the thought that after that he'll have to deal with a hard-on in a room full of other academics for the rest of the day."

"I have a hard-on-in-the-office problem myself," I told her.

"Why's that?" she said almost shyly. "Is there a particular workmate who causes it?"

"Just some new bimbo." I laughed.

"Bimbo! That's it, I'm hanging up." But she didn't and then laughed with me.

"Send him a text now. Tell him you're rubbing yourself under your desk."

"I like it. Then what?"

"Imagine me there . . . under your desk . . . touching and licking."

"You're so naughty," she said, but I knew she'd be doing it soon.

"I try to be," I said smarmily.

"It's working."

"Good. When you have the picture in your mind, reach down under your desk. Rub yourself through your clothes."

I heard her suck in her breath sharply, and I knew she'd started.

"I'm walking down," I said, and hung up before she could protest.

By the time I got to her office, she'd zipped up and, though looking a bit flushed, was composed and professional.

She grinned and told me to close the door.

"Yes, ma'am."

She suddenly looked a little serious.

"Cheryl or someone is going to catch us if we keep this up," she said.

"Catch what?" I smiled and crossed to her desk. Resting on the edge, my crotch was just a couple of feet from her face as she remained seated.

"What am I going to do with you?" She grinned.

"Whatever you can think of," I said, wiggling my eyebrows in my lousy Groucho impression.

"That sounds like it might be fun," she said.

"Could be very fun," I said, and offered her my hand.

She took it and stood, and with my knees parted slightly she had no choice but to position herself between them. She did, however, remain a good three feet away.

"But no kissing," I chuckled, repeating the first law she'd laid down to me.

"You like kisses." It was a statement, not a question, and I saw something in her eyes that hadn't been there before.

"Yes, I do, Lu. Do you like kisses?"

"Yes," she said very quietly, dropping her gaze from mine.

Taking a chance, I cupped her face and turned it upward, at the same time pulling her forward.

"What are we up to, Lu?"

"Well, I'm trying to get out of here to meet my kids before the school bus dumps them by the front door," she said, still not pulling away.

I leaned in and whispered in her ear, knowing my breath was tickling her.

"Ahhh, I see. How about a kiss before you go?"

She hesitated for a second and then thrilled me by saying it.

"Okay—one kiss."

I wrapped my arms around her and pulled her tight enough for her to feel how hard I was.

"That feels nice," Lu whispered.

"So will this," I said, and I began to kiss her neck, her ears, her throat. I ran my hands up and down her back.

Her lips parted slightly, but before she could speak, I pulled her even tighter and covered her mouth with mine.

She shivered and began to rock slightly against my erection. She broke the kiss, but only to nibble my neck and earlobe, and I squeezed and kneaded the delectable ass that had first caught my eye.

Our mouths collided again in a hungry open-mouth kiss. Our tongues were dueling, sliding in and out of each other's mouths, our breath ragged and coming in gasps.

With one hand still caressing her ass, I tangled the other in her hair. It's a tired cliché, but I locked on to her mouth like a drowning man holds on to a life preserver.

"I'm in trouble—I'm on fire," Lu whispered fiercely.

"And you have to go," I said, and again covered her mouth with mine to block her answer.

The kiss lingered, but when it broke, we were both smiling.

"Go, Lu," I said. "Be good."

"How?" She laughed and pushed me away.

She pulled me close again, though, and I could see fire in her eyes as she stared up at me.

"See you tomorrow, Lu."

"I know—and that's the problem. I'll be stuck here playing teasing games with you, and I won't be getting any at home for the next seven days." But she was still smiling as she watched me back toward the door and out of her office.

The real problem, though, was the call I got when I settled back in behind my desk. My wife's cell phone came up on the caller ID.

"Hey, babe, what's up?" I asked.

"Just wanted to remind you that I'm taking the kids to the beach for the weekend tomorrow."

That was when it hit me. Lu's husband was gone for a week. Me alone for the weekend—because Lu and I were working all weekend. With probably no one else in the office . . .

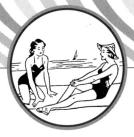

GUITAR FREAKOUT

J. M. Thompson

Sandy and Tammy could still hear the faint strains of the guitars on the beach as a few of their friends were butchering the Ventures' "Walk Don't Run." They had done a decent job with "Pipeline," but somehow without the beat of the drum driving the rhythm, they just weren't making it happen.

"Do you think they know anything else, or will they keep killing that song?" Tammy asked.

"Yeah, it's a real guitar freakout. Actually, I'm kind of glad they only know those two songs. I'd hate to see them destroy something really good like the Beach Boys or something."

"Or a Paul Revere & the Raiders," Tammy replied.

"Oh, you're just nuts about Mark Lindsay."

"What about Fang?"

"Oh, come on, Tammy. Fang just plays guitar, and I've see you drooling over Mark," Sandy said.

"Yeah, he is dreamy, but guys aren't like that. That's why . . ." She didn't finish.

Sitting down next to Tammy, Sandy put her arm around her friend. She wanted to finish what she had said but didn't want to make things uncomfortable. They had seemed to be drawing closer and closer together as they watched their friends pair up into couples and start dating. Now, after wandering away from the group on the beach, they found themselves alone in one of the beach shacks the surfers often used.

Turning her head a bit, Sandy kissed Tammy on the cheek, and as her friend slowly turned her head too, they kissed, lightly at first, but then Sandy slipped her tongue into Tammy's mouth. They had kissed before, but they had been quick kisses stolen in the moments when their other friends were looking away. Now they just kissed, both frightened but excited.

Sandy continued kissing Tammy, their tongues sliding between each other's lips, while moving her hand up inside Tammy's blouse. Sliding it up over top of her bathing suit, she squeezed lightly, and when Tammy didn't pull away, she moved her hand under her friend's top, feeling a nipple slide between her fingers.

"Should we be doing this?" Tammy asked. "They may come looking for us. I mean, the music stopped."

"If the music stopped, then they are probably doing exactly what we're doing."

"What are we doing?"

"We are doing something that feels right. It feels right, doesn't it?" Sandy asked.

"Yes," Tammy answered, backing away from Sandy as she unbuttoned her blouse and then pulled off the top of her bathing suit. She paused, waiting for Sandy to do the same. Then they embraced, feeling their naked breasts brush against each other. Pulling apart, they playfully pushed out their breasts, touching nipples. Finally, Sandy leaned forward and slid her mouth over one of Tammy's nipples, sucking it lightly while running the palm of her hand over her other one.

Tammy leaned back on the cot as Sandy remained on top of her, sucking and licking her nipples while moving her thigh between Tammy's legs. Hearing her friend breathing heavily, Sandy continued, lightly squeezing Tammy's breasts while moving her hips and grinding herself against Tammy's thigh while she pushed her thigh against her. When Tammy lifted her hips, pushing back against Sandy, she quickened her pace, feeling the pleasure running through her body.

They continued grinding against each other as Sandy rose up and stared into her friend's eyes. Somehow they both knew this was exactly what each wanted, exactly what they had been searching for throughout all those dates in high school, the seemingly pointless fumbling with the boys. Now, with both about to head off to college, they were discovering something, something they seemed to have been searching for for almost nineteen years.

Feeling the pleasure overtake her, Sandy moaned loudly and said, "Oh, Tammy," as she came, pressing against her friend's thigh.

Sandy stopped moving, but then Tammy pleaded, "Please don't stop, I'm almost . . ."

Sandy pressed against her friend, leaning a bit on her thigh as she ground against her. Tammy responded by lifting her hips, actually raising Sandy off the cot a bit. Tammy then closed her eyes and fell back onto the cot, gasping. Opening her eyes, she grabbed her friend's head and pulled it down to her, where they locked in a kiss.

After a few minutes, Tammy broke the silence, whispering, "Sandy, I didn't know it could be like that."

"I thought I knew what it would be like. I mean, I felt something with some of the boys when we messed around, but, well, this is so different."

"I hear music," Tammy suddenly said, sitting up straight.

"We'd better be getting back," Sandy said, handing Tammy her top. "I can't wait until next week. I'm going to miss you."

"But I'll be right there with you."

"We'll be together, but not like this, not like we want," Sandy replied.

Touching her lover's cheek, Tammy said, "Just be patient. One day, one day we will." She leaned forward and kissed Sandy on the forehead. "We better get going."

They both quickly pulled on their bikini tops and blouses and then peeked out of the shack. No one was around, so they slipped out the door and then walked back toward the group on the beach.

"They must have the radio on because that's real music I hear," Sandy said.

Wandering back into their group of friends, Sandy sat on the other side of the fire from Tammy. The others were all sitting together in couples, singing to the songs on the radio. Tammy heard it first, the chimes at the beginning of the song, and as the radio played "Cherish" by The Association, she looked over to Sandy.

Staring into each other's eyes, they sang, *"Cherish is the word I use to describe all the feelings that I have hiding here for you inside."*

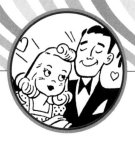

MEMORY LANE

C. M. Bradley

It was a Thursday. I remember because it was the first day of the month. I received a call from my old girlfriend Tina. I called her T for short. It was a private joke because the first time I met her she was wearing a wet T-shirt with no bra. Yeah, I was in love. T was my first love. I was at the tender age of seventeen and a whole year older than her. We had lost our virginities to each other. Wow, that was a day to remember. She placed herself in my skillful hands since I was older and the male. Sure, as if I knew what I was doing. I was a graduate of BU (Bullshit University) with a master's degree in gullible from listening to my freak friends, who obtained their unreliable information from older relatives. After countless days of dry humping and fumbling with each other, it finally happened. I felt like such a man. Despite ejaculating into a condom, it was the first time I had ejaculated with someone other than me in the room. I still remember her naked body as if it were yesterday. Damn, her ass always looked good.

Anyway, she called to inform me that she was going to be in my area for a business meeting and wanted to have dinner. Myriad emotions overcame me. It was all I could do to agree and get the date when she would be in town.

The day had finally arrived, and I was in the shower getting ready for the big event. It had been twenty years since we had seen each other. What would happen? How much had she changed? Would there still be a special bond between us? I had so many questions. As I stood there in front of the mirror drying myself, I looked at the changes that had occurred in me. An obvious one was the beer gut I had been perfecting. Another one was my incredibly shrinking penis. I remember how big both my heads got when T expressed fear after seeing my erect penis for the first time. The only emotion my penis could evoke now was laughter. I guess it wasn't too bad when it was erect. Hell, now my ego was getting the better of me. In any event, what in the world would possess me to think I would have anything other than a delicious meal and good conversation? I put on my best "I'm still cool" clothes and headed to the restaurant.

I arrived a few minutes early. I counted that as a check in the excellent block of my mental report card. It was my understanding that the restaurant was a few blocks from her hotel. Would she walk or drive? What did I care? With my luck, I'd be the one sitting in the restaurant watching my car getting the business end of a tow truck. Just then, in she came. She looked relatively the same as she had twenty years ago. Her smile lit up the room when she recognized me. I couldn't help but give her a kiss on the cheek and step back. We looked at each other, and I was amazed at how good she looked. I could only imagine what she was thinking about me. We spent a few moments with introductory chatter and then were escorted to our table. I helped her with her coat, and the whiff of perfume made me want to just drop the coat and start nibbling on her neck. Her outfit complemented her figure and was quite classy. We sat, and the conversation was as fluid as if a day had never passed. I was on my best behavior and trying very hard to be charming. I built up enough nerve to ask about any possible relationships. That was when the waiter decided to walk up and take our order. His tip had just taken a turn for the worse. I placed another favorable check on my report card by ordering the drinks and meal for both of us. As the waiter stepped away, T began a funny anecdote about the last time she had that meal. *Come on, cut to the chase. I'm going to laugh regardless of what happened.* I wanted to get back to the conversation about relationships.

She knew what I wanted to talk about because after her anecdote, her voice and head dropped. In a soft voice, I informed her that we could talk about anything. T then explained that she recently had finalized her divorce. She had come to realize that her ex was never going to grow up and thought she should end it before they became enemies. She further explained that the divorce was amicable and that she was over it. I then asked about previous love interests. It appeared they were few and far between. She was like most business-oriented women, and her sex life had suffered while she was climbing the ladder of success. Our meal arrived, and more jovial topics prevailed. The coy eye contact and cheeky smiles were a little uncomfortable, but we were both taking it well. The meal was just about done, and somehow the status of my relationships finally came up. Would the truth really work in this situation? Did she really need to hear the truth? For her "own good," I decided to skirt the truth and tell her what she wanted to hear. It just so happened that what I told her made me available for sex if she felt so inclined.

The meal was done, and I helped her with her coat. We exited the restaurant and stood outside for a few minutes talking. When it appeared we were done, I kissed T on the cheek. The pause and eye contact afterward begged for something more. I then gave her a tender kiss on the lips. I could feel her moist lips kissing me back. I asked her how she was getting back to her hotel. She said she had walked. I certainly could not allow her to walk back alone, and so the slow stroll toward ecstasy began. The street was quiet, and it was beginning to drizzle. We walked, looked in the store windows, and talked about life. A life when things were simpler. Like when we were teenagers. And there we were, right where I wanted to be. At her hotel and talking about sexual encounters. The drizzle slowly picked up to a solid rain. At least the weather was on my side. As if she were reading my mind, T invited me up until it stopped raining. As I was walking through the lobby and stepping into the elevator, I knew I was crossing the line. As we were going up in the elevator, you could cut the tension with a knife. The conversation became strained. Should I excuse myself? I could feel the brain center in my pants setting up shop, and the signals from the big head were shutting down.

We exited the elevator and were walking toward her room. I could feel that my clothes and face were damp, but my mind was focused on looking at her ass swish back and forth beneath her coat. We entered the luxury room, and I was impressed. "Very nice," I muttered. My mind was struggling for something intelligent or witty to say. As she threw me a towel, I took off my coat and shoes. She suggested that I turn on the television while she got comfortable. I found something mildly entertaining to watch and stretched out across the bed. Then I heard the shower running. Should the shower be running? Was she actually going to get naked with me roaming through the room? Good Lord, was there a chapter in *Dating for Dummies* that dealt with this kind of situation? I didn't know what else to do but wait for her next move.

She came out of the bathroom wearing a robe, a towel on her hair, and carrying a bottle of baby oil. She sat on the edge of the bed, opened the baby oil, and started rubbing it on her feet. Being a gentleman, I insisted that she sit back and allow me to take care of that for her. After all, it had been a fantastic evening thus far and it was all due to her. The mental report card just received another excellent check. She agreed and sat back against the headboard. During her shifting, her robe came open slightly and I could see that she had on only a pair of panties. The erotic visions were rampantly running through my mind. I poured some baby oil into the palm of my hand and began an erotic massage on one foot. I knew that once my oily fingers passed through her perfectly shaped toes, something was going to happen. As sensually as I could, I rubbed the oil onto her foot and up her calf. In addition to her inhibitions, her topic of conversation relaxed. T then informed me that since "us," no man had ever treated her with such tenderness. Despite accumulating some skills with regard to sex, she still embraced our awkward encounters. My concern for her needs and pleasure had never been duplicated or replaced. I felt a bashful smile envelop my face. Luckily, her eyes were closed and her head tilted back because I felt at that moment that I was unable to look her in the eye. I merely thanked her for the comment and poured more oil for the other foot. I didn't think it was possible, but my skill level for erotic massage rose along with my penis and her robe. I found my oil-rich hands sliding above the knee and heading for the upper thigh. I felt her legs opening, allowing me access. As my hand brushed against her panties, I could feel heat and moisture. Unless one of us came to our senses, it was going to happen.

I decided to give her an opportunity to cease our course of action by standing and removing my shirt. Instead, she used that moment to remove her robe and help me with my pants. As she pulled my boxers down for me, she came face to face with a part of my anatomy that she hadn't seen in two decades. She took my package into her hands and carefully pushed back my pubic hair. Her mouth opened, and she used her tongue like a shoehorn to slowly insert my cock into her mouth. This was a skill that had improved since last we met. She teased and sucked me to full length and stopped to admire her work.

"This is the dick that started it all," she said.

The fact that she wasn't laughing and shooting snot from her nose was a victory for me. I looked at her body and just wanted to cherish it before I ravished it. So I asked her if she would allow me to finish my massage.

She looked at me and said, "If that's what you want to do, fine."

She slid back onto the bed and offered herself to me. I grabbed the oil and finished her legs and began on her arms. While touching her body I was finding it hard to put more than two words together between gulps. Completing sentences was totally out of the question. When I finished her arms, I placed a small amount of oil on her stomach and began small circles until I reached her breasts. Normally, I preferred larger breasts, but in her case I was more than willing to make an exception. With each slow pass of her nipples, each of us released a low moan.

Realizing that I needed to catch my breath, I asked her to roll over. That was truly a mistake. I hadn't discovered until that moment that she was wearing a thong. The sight of those magnificent butt cheeks in that thong would have caused a coronary in a weaker man. I collected myself along with the bottle of oil and continued my task. I started with her back because I knew touching that apple bottom would have to be last. While I massaged her back, she continued to lament about our last sexual encounters. I knew that they had meant a lot to me, but I was never aware of the impact they had on her. By the time I reached her buttocks, I was compelled to reveal my unrelenting desire to touch her ass. She laughed and recalled the many times in our youth I palmed her ass while playing and especially during sex. She knew I just couldn't keep my hands off her ass. She said that was probably why she started wearing thongs. I could no longer resist. I slipped my fingers under the waistband of the thong and slowly pulled it down. Watching the garment pop out of the crack of her ass was a bonus. She rolled over, and our eyes met. I lowered my body onto hers, supporting my weight with my arms. Our kiss was a passionate one that contained many messages of desire. Then T reminded me of the time I tried to fuck her tits. That was truly a sad attempt, but since we were just learning, it wasn't as devastating as it could have been. T said she knew how much I loved large breasts and that I must have completed that act with someone. She wanted to give me that opportunity again.

She reached for the oil and rubbed some across her chest. Using her oily hand, she stroked my cock to a full and throbbing mass. She lay back and asked me to straddle her. Her breasts were not ample enough to wrap around my cock, but their appearance was quite capable of keeping me erect. She rested the heel of her palm on one and placed her fingertips on the other, leaving a space for me to slide my cock under her hand. I grabbed on to the headboard and hung on for the ride. I closed my eyes and made love to her hand and chest. The sensation of my nut sack dragging across her chest was mind-shattering. The oil and her hand were working like a charm. The occasional glimpse of her face and nipples brought me to my peak. I felt the end was close. My pace slowed, my heart raced, and my moans grew louder. At the moment of explosion, she placed a firm grip on my cock and pointed it toward the underside of her chin. I opened my eyes in time to see the first load deflect off her chin. The second and third streams weren't as strong and dribbled across her chest but were just as satisfying. As my juices began to pool into a notch in her neck, she pulled me toward her mouth. I inched forward and tilted my body so that she could squeeze the remaining droplets onto her outstretched tongue. From the look on her face, I couldn't tell which one of us enjoyed it more.

After a brief stint of unconsciousness caused by an excess amount of ecstasy, my hands began exploring her soft curves. I didn't know if or when I would get another opportunity like that, so I had to admire that booty one last time. As I picked up the baby oil from the floor, I coaxed her to roll onto her stomach. I held the bottle so that the oil would drip out onto her sexy mounds. The droplets slowly ran off the mounds in every direction. My widespread fingers savored every inch as I massaged the oil into her skin. My hands loved the splendid symmetry of her soft, plump hindquarters. My thumbs came together at the point where her inner thighs and butt cheeks met. They dug into the folds of the skin and slid upward into the split of her ass. I paused momentarily to explore the edges of her anal opening. The low moan indicated that the action needed to be repeated. This time when I stopped on the rim of her anal opening, I carefully inserted both thumbs into her. From the relaxed response, I could tell this action was not foreign to her. I teased, twisted, and tugged the sphincter muscle until I could fully insert both thumbs. I was so focused on what I was doing that I failed to notice that her breathing was labored and her pleasure was peaking. I thought I was being suggestive and/or talking dirty when I said, "You really need my dick in your ass."

I was shocked at the response: "What are you waiting for?"

On that note, I decided to terminate my half-assed proctology exam. I pulled my thumbs out one at a time, stood up, and thoroughly oiled my cock. T positioned herself as if she had done this before while being tied to the bed. Her legs and arms were pointed to each corner of the bed and slightly squirming. From a kneeling position, I propped myself up with one hand while using the oily hand to place the tip of my cock on her backdoor. As the head penetrated, she reached back with both hands and spread her butt cheeks as far as possible. Little by little my cock disappeared into her. Her grunts concerned me but were quickly dispelled when I heard, "Fuck me." Once I was fully inserted, I supported my upper body with my fully extended arms and hands. The middle of my torso was grinding on her plump ass with each downstroke. I could feel her sphincter muscle constricting around my throbbing tool on the upstroke and my pubic hairs rubbing against her ass on the downstroke. As we pounded again and again, there was no doubt our lust could be heard in the adjacent rooms. When I heard her reaching her climax, I pushed down as hard and deep as I could. I slowed my pace and rotated my hips until she could catch her breath. The complete submission and surrender of her body to me was utterly fantastic. Once we were both ready, I picked up the pace until we both peaked at the same time.

There wasn't much left, but I could feel the surge from my balls go through my cock and leak out of the tip as it came to rest deep within her. Withdrawing my manhood and watching it dangle and drip onto her ass was very different from anything we had ever done.

I rolled onto the bed beside her and stared at the ceiling. I was reveling in the sensations flowing through my cock and feeling the sweat drying on my body. T rolled onto her side and commented on how much better we both had become at sex. She snuggled up close and started playing with the hair on my chest. I put my arm around her and stroked her soft skin. We just lay there and reminisced about the old days well into the night. I didn't want to leave until she mentioned she had to get up at seven for a meeting. I got up and took a quick shower. When I exited the bathroom, T was curled up and asleep on the bed with the blankets at her feet. I covered her up, dressed, and left a note requesting that she call me whenever she wanted. I gave her a light kiss on the forehead and slipped out undetected. The walk back to my car through the mist just couldn't last long enough. It was unfortunate that my mental report card and any other evidence would have to be destroyed before I got home.

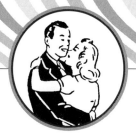

No Coincidence

Anne Alexander

There he was again, standing downstairs in the crowd, watching the band, his face illuminated. It was the third time in a month she'd seen him at this club, and she was starting to think maybe it wasn't a coincidence. She looked away for a minute, pretending to scan the crowd behind her for the friends who were supposed to meet her there. When she looked back, he was looking at her. Her heart leaped in her chest, and she smiled at him. He smiled back.

Well, she thought, *this is how it all went before, too. I wonder if we'll ever talk to each other. Do I have to make the first move?*

So she did. She looked down from her spot on the balcony and waved, making it clear it was to him she was beckoning. He waved back, and she smiled again. The band launched into a faster song, one she always turned up and danced to in her kitchen.

She started dancing now, moving her hips and flipping her hair, letting her eyes lock on his every once in a while. She raised her arms above her head and moved them, too. The next time she looked at him, his gaze was fixed on her. He was mesmerized. She felt amazingly sexy, dancing for him, so she kept going faster and faster as he watched. And even though the club was pretty packed, she felt like they were the only two people there.

The song ended, and she clapped and screamed for the band. As she glanced down at her mystery man, he was clapping too, but he was still looking up at her. She got a little embarrassed then and tried to compose herself. She turned her attention back to the band, which was getting into a slow, soulful song. She took a deep breath, then looked back down to where he was.

But he wasn't there anymore. She scanned the crowd, trying to make him out, but she couldn't see him. Damn, she thought.

"Damn. I blew it," she said aloud to herself.

"Nah, I don't think so. You've still got a shot," a voice behind her said right into her ear.

She whirled around, and of course it was he. "Hi!" she said, slightly sheepish at being caught talking to herself but glad to be face to face with her mystery man after so much prolonged flirting from afar.

"Hi. I'm—"

"No, wait, don't tell me yet. Keep it a secret," she said, turning back around and resting her hands on the railing of the balcony. She reached behind her and caught each of his hands in hers and brought them around her, putting his hands on the railing with hers. He was right up against her now.

It's pretty dark up here, she thought. A fair amount of people, too. I wonder how much I can get away with. . . .

She began to sway her hips to the music, and she moved her hands so that they were over his and caressed them lightly. She could feel the front of his jeans through the thin material of her skirt, and she was glad she'd worn it instead of jeans. Glad it was warm enough to forgo tights, too.

"What are you up to?" he whispered into her ear. She reached up and touched his cheek, holding him there by her face. His was slightly rough with stubble, and she liked it. She turned her head to kiss him quickly on the cheek, but he turned his head fast and caught her with his lips. She was surprised at first but then melted into it, opening her mouth slightly and letting his tongue in to touch hers. It was a soft, sweet kiss, but it got faster and more urgent quickly, until she was sucking on his bottom lip and he was nipping lightly at hers. She could feel the urgency elsewhere, too, as the hardness under his jeans grew and she rubbed her ass against him.

"Just getting to know you," she whispered back, letting the tip of her tongue flick into his ear. She felt him gasp.

"You're killing me," he groaned, finding her lips with his again and kissing her hard. He was grinding himself into her backside now, and she took his left hand and brought it under her jacket, up her body and to her breast.

He didn't resist. Instead, he moved to her nipple and pinched it between his thumb and finger. It was her turn to gasp as she felt the liquid fire feeling melt through her and down between her legs.

"Oh!" she cried out as he circled his finger around her taut nipple.

He giggled into her ear, loving the effect he was having on her, this beautiful stranger. She turned sharply toward him, but before she could reprimand him for laughing at her, he caught her mouth with his again, running his tongue over her bottom lip and effectively silencing her for the moment. He trailed his lips down her neck, kissing around it and up to her ear. She thought she would go crazy with the sensations she was feeling—she was sure she wouldn't be able to stand much more of this without having him inside her.

The band revved up after yet another slow jam, beginning its one minor hit, and the crowd was into it again.

She sought out his ear. "I have to have you. Now." As she spoke, she reached behind her and found his zipper. She rubbed his cock on the inside of his jeans for a moment, then unzipped and reached in. He took a sharp breath.

"Wait, wait," he begged. "We can just go somewhere . . . back to my place . . . I only live a couple of blocks from here." But as he whispered into her ear, his penis grew harder in her hand, and she was sure she could talk him into staying right where they were.

"But I really like this band," she told him, a grin playing on the edges of her mouth.

He groaned again. "Have it your way," he said as his left hand continued playing expertly with her nipple. His right hand, meanwhile, reached between their bodies and under her short skirt. He was thrilled to find only a silky strip of thong there, and he quickly moved it aside.

"Ohhhhh," she purred as his fingers found what they were looking for. "Ohhh!"

"You like that?" he asked, eliciting a few more moans. He kept going, circling his fingers in her wet center, then moving up to the sensitive spot right above, then back again.

"Yes," she whispered, continuing to rub his cock. "I wish I could suck you now," she told him, "but I think that might blow our cover!" She laughed at her own silly joke, then gave in again to the sensations he was providing.

The band finished its hit, and the crowd applauded. She stopped, and he stopped, and they both clapped loudly and hooted as the band launched into another peppy, poppy song.

She found his ear. "Condom," she said. "Now."

"Yeah, I have one. Right here."

"Hurry."

"Yes, okay . . . here we go, okay. . . . It's on. You're sure I can't convince you to go back—"

She reached behind her and grabbed his penis, making sure it was covered, and turned her head. She kissed him again and then found his ear with her lips. "Do it. Now." She got on her tiptoes as he squatted a bit, finding the right angle. Then he thrust himself into her, slowly for the first couple of inches, then ramming himself all the way in. "Ohhhhhh," she moaned. "Yes, that's good. . . ."

"Yeah? Yeah? It's good?" he spoke right into her ear as he thrust into her again and again, feeling her warm wetness and his own resolve to keep going forever weaken. He reached around and rubbed her sweet spot through her skirt.

"It's so good. So good. Go faster. I'm so close. So close."

He sped up, wanting to savor the feeling of her but not able to keep his composure as the band reached a crescendo in the song. The crowd around them sang at the top of their lungs and moved to the music as he pumped into her again and again and she whimpered that she was coming, "Slow down, I'm coming," she said, trying not to shout as his fingers found just the right tempo and he slowed his thrusts. She felt it build, build, build, and then suddenly a shower of stars and she was there. "Ohhhhh . . ." She trailed off, feeling that she might not be able to stand up for much longer.

But he had her in his arms, the song was coming to its climax, and the contractions inside her had their effect on him and he was shooting his load inside her. It felt so good. "So good," he moaned, "so, so, so good," feeling the last spasms as he slowed down and stopped thrusting, kissing her neck and stroking her belly as they both quieted down and the song ended.

The crowd clapped and hollered; this was the end of the set! He withdrew from her and zipped up as she straightened her skirt, then they both clapped and yelled for an encore from the band. "WOOOO," they screamed, laughing and applauding.

She felt fantastic. She looked back at him and smiled broadly. "Okay, now tell me your name."

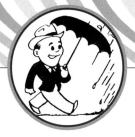

A PERFECT STORM

Nancy Brophy

We are seated in the bar, a funky gothic place with red velvet drapes covering the door to keep the cool fall breeze outside as people come and go. The drink menu is suitably intriguing for our tastes, and we toy between caipirinhas or caprioskas and choose the former, deciding that our last foray into the evil of cachaça has left us willing to go there again. We have been huddled against the menu, canoodling, so absorbed in our task that we do not realize that others have been watching us and speculating. After we get our luscious drinks and began sipping, the woman on the bar stool next to me leans over and asks if we are on a first date. We cannot help but giggle as we gaze into each other's eyes as we have done so many times while doing such wicked things to each other.

"Oh, no," you reply with your sweet grin tugging at your handsome face, your eyes practically dancing with mischief. I have seen that look so many times before and feel the thin strip of satin between my bare thighs go moist with your words. We chat with the couple beside us, who ironically are on a first date, and another couple, but ultimately get lost in each other, as we are wont to do. You look so handsome, having dressed for me this evening, taking pride in selecting the perfect outfit to accompany your natural beauty. Your skin is so smooth, and I run the back of my fingers down your chiseled cheek to your chin with its distinctive cleft, your eyes twinkling above your strong nose as your seductive lips slowly spread into a smile at my touch.

I lean in for a kiss and can smell the Burberry cologne on your skin, so soft for such a masculine man, such broad shoulders and strong arms that I know can manipulate me to the most sinful of predicaments. And to think they thought we were on a first date. If only they could read our minds. . . . I see the wind whipping the trees through the windows across the street; it is the perfect fall evening: dark, mysterious, and I am feeling the seductive pull of my cocktail and your body near mine.

The weather has gotten even worse when we leave the bar, and we scamper for your car, huddling against the wind. Back at our place, we scramble up the stairs, out of breath and pulling at each other's clothes, invigorated by the wind whipping around us as we rush in the door. The heat of your kiss warms me, as do your fingers along my bare thighs, seeking my center, confirming that I have been desperate to have you for the past hour as we sat making idle chitchat and being respectable in public. There is not much respectable about us behind closed doors.

You tug my jacket off, getting locks of my long blond hair caught in the process, exposing my throat. You take advantage and lean in, devouring me with your lips, your teeth gently nipping at my neck, my ears, eliciting moans of bliss. You flick the button to my little cardigan, roughly shoving it off my shoulders, pull my camisole down, and squeeze my breasts together, biting my now-hard nipples through my bra. Wanting more flesh, we fight each other to expose my skin, then I need yours, and I begin undoing the buttons covering your glorious chest. You are an Adonis, your smooth skin taut over such perfect muscles that I shiver touching you.

I continue my journey south, relieving your beautiful manhood of the constraints of your trousers, dropping to my knees to engulf you in the hot wetness of my mouth. I am so desperate to taste you, feel you, that I try to swallow every bit of you that I can, taking you to the depths of my throat. I remain there for a moment, feeling your pulse with my own, beating as one: mutual desire. I slowly withdraw, feeling your thickness between my lips, savoring the sensation as I use the tip of my tongue to caress the underside of your beautiful cock. I reach your thick head and swirl around and around, gently probing for any sweet precome, and my ministrations are generously rewarded with a drop of the juice we both savor so much. I slide my hands around to your glutes, spreading my palms across your cheeks and squeezing, loving the feel of your ass in my hands. I gently pull your cheeks apart, slide one hand in, and tickle your rosebud and taint with my finger and am rewarded with a moan from you and a slight trembling in your knees.

You pull me up abruptly, unzipping my skirt and pushing me over the easy chair behind me. My legs are splayed, and I am at your mercy. You know this as you dive into my bare center, hitting my hard clit right away, but only to tease for a bit before licking lower, between my lips, gently tugging with your teeth, sucking my nectar. You return to my clit, alternately licking, flicking, and gently biting, adding your thick fingers to my slick opening as you ravage me. I am soon writhing on the chair, not sure if I am trying to have you or get away from such exquisite pleasure, but soon enough I cry out.

"Oh, Dominic, oh, I'm coming, Baby, don't stop!" I buck against your hand, your lips, as wave after wave rushes through me, and every muscle in my body contracts. You continue to suckle me as the intensity of my orgasm ebbs, your gaze locked onto mine as your fingers find mine and intertwine.

You climb up my body, biting a hard nipple in a way that tells me you are in no mood for cuddling but need release. Just at that moment, the wind whips against the skylights in a fierce gust, and we are both momentarily distracted. We get up and move to the couch, drawn by the storm that appears to be escalating outside as much as in our home. We pull a throw around our shoulders and watch as the storm rolls across the ocean; it is picturesque in the night. After a few moments of this, it is almost as if we have the same thought at the same time.

We toss the blanket aside and head out onto the deck, completely oblivious to the temperature in the fifties. We are a bit worried about the neighbors at first despite the late hour and stay close to the side of the house, you pinning me against the side with your warmth as you kiss me passionately. We are surrounded by wind, whipping our skin, my hair, the smell of the ocean as it churns. Your kisses deepen, and soon you are turning me around and I am grasping the railing of the deck as you enter me from behind. I have a momentary thought of the neighbors, the house across the driveway, and the windows at eye level with me at this moment, but I just don't care as your thickness slides into me to the hilt.

I grip the railing even tighter, feeling every bit of you in that first thrust, your hips flush with mine before you withdraw and slam home again. There is nothing tender tonight; our passion is as fierce as the wind howling around us. A flash of lightning illuminates the sky as you hammer into me. I can almost see the white of my knuckles gripping the railing. I'm not sure if it's from holding on or from pushing back onto you as you slam into me. I can't seem to take you deep enough, am as wild as the waves churning against the breakwater across the street. You lean forward, cupping my breasts, so that now you are flush with me as you slide in and out in smooth, well-aimed movements that hit all the right spots. I am almost hanging over the railing at this point, unaware of the turmoil brewing around us.

You pull back and guide me to a chair, seating me and pulling me so my ass is barely on the edge, as am I at this point. You slide your iron-hard rod into me for a moment; my eyes start to roll into the back of my head, but you have so much more in store for me. More flashes of lightning are glistening across the bay, reflecting in your eyes, and there are now rumbles of thunder as you position the head of your thick cock at my little knot. It is cold outside, and my flesh is goose-pimpled; my body automatically contracts with the cold, yet I feel the heat of you at my backdoor, and my legs splay just a bit more to grant access.

You begin to push, and I feel the crown sliding in, that initial ease before the inevitable pop when the head completely violates my most decadent space. Is there any more delicious feeling? You pull my ankles up as you simultaneously slide deeper into my ass, then, with one final thrust, you are buried balls-deep. You know how much I love it when you wait there a moment, and despite the growing mayhem swirling around us, you manage to thrust just a bit deeper, then swirl your hips, driving me absolutely mad with desire. I reach up and pinch your already hard nipples, gently tugging as you slam into my ass, holding my ankles up and apart, taking my ass so completely. Your thrusts are wild, deep, and strong as you fill me in the way only you know that I love. I am pinned against the back of the deck chair, barely able to meet your thrusts, but I clench my ass, gripping you, trying to keep you as deep inside me as possible, feeling every bit of you as you hammer in and out of my tight ass.

Our moans become deafening, and even with the growing thunderclaps I am sure our neighbors must be able to hear something. But at this point, I just don't care. All I care about is your thick cock sliding in and out of my tight knot as wind and thunder swirl around us, and I look up to the cacophony of tree branches dancing overhead with my ankles in my periphery. Just as I am about to lose total control, I feel a cool droplet on my chest. And then another. Suddenly, there is torrential rain pouring down on us, but this seems perfect for the moment. I find myself falling over the edge, crying out in ecstasy as I come and come, feel you growing even more rigid in my ass, slamming into me, then pausing, only to thrust one final time before releasing my ankles as your body grows rigid with your final thrust. I feel hot torrents erupt into me as cool rain splatters onto us, see you arched in ecstasy in a flash of lightning before you collapse over me. Your heart is thumping against mine as thunder roars around us, rain beats down on your back, rolling off you and onto me, our bodies still joined and spent.

After a few moments, the coldness overwhelms us, and we scamper, shivering, into the house. I draw a hot shower and lead you into the steam, wrapping you in my arms as we collapse against each other, using the wall for support. We stay under the steam long enough to warm our shivering bodies, then wrap into towels with our wrinkled skin and amazed looks before climbing into bed, still catching each other's glances in the streaks of lightning across the sky as we lay under the skylight: the calm after a perfect storm.

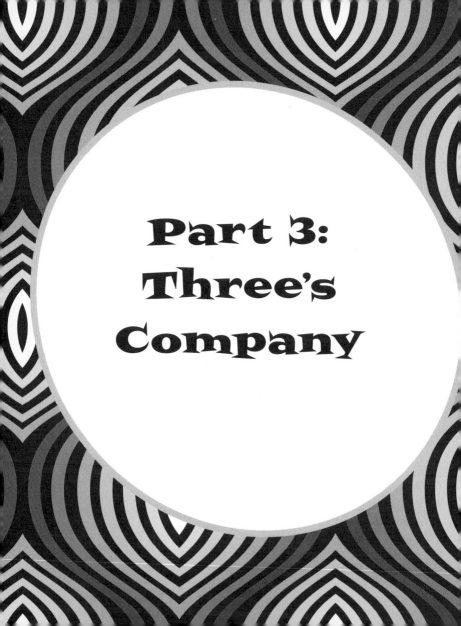

Part 3: Three's Company

The only unnatural sex act is that
which you cannot perform.

—Dr. Alfred Kinsey

Now that you're pretty well versed in one-on-one sex, why not add another person, right? Well, that's up to you and your partner, of course. Lots of folks love the idea of a threesome and fantasize about it but wouldn't actually want to realize that fantasy. Then there are those who love the idea and the actuality, those who want to experience sex with two people at once and are looking to make that happen. This part of the book is for them. But before we explore the ins and outs and dos and don'ts, we need to define some terms so that the rest of this section makes verbal sense to you even if the impetus behind threesomes remains confusingly opaque.

THREESOME GLOSSARY

* **ALTERNATIVE LIFESTYLE:** Generic term for anything considered outside the "normal" realm of sexual behavior from spankings and shoe fetishes to threesomes and key parties.

* **BISEXUAL:** Used to describe a person who is sexually attracted to and has sex with men and women. Behavioral psychologists and sex experts alike talk about continua, scales, and actual attraction, but we needn't concern ourselves with scientific discussions of "true" bisexuality. Suffice it to say that for our purposes, "bi" means interested in sleeping with both sexes.

* **BICURIOUS:** Describes a person who is interested in exploring and maybe even experiencing same-sex behavior but doesn't necessarily identify as bisexual.

* **COMPERSION:** The feeling of pleasure one gets when one's partner is having sex with someone else; the opposite of jealousy.

* **CUCKOLD:** Almost an open marriage; this scenario occurs when one partner has sex with an outside person and then shares the details with the other partner.

STRETCHING THE TRUTH

Historically, the word *cuckold* referred to a husband whose wife was cheating on him. It's been around since the 1200s, although we're sure the practice is a lot older.

* **DOUBLE PENETRATION:** In a threesome with two men and a woman, this term describes both men having intercourse with the woman, usually one vaginally and one anally.
* **MÉNAGE À TROIS:** Not synonymous with "threesome"; actually describes three people in a love relationship together.

COMMUNICATION

Ménage à trois is a French term. What a surprise.

* **SOFT SWING:** Generally refers to threesome practices in which you don't engage in penetration with anyone but your long-term partner; this may mean oral sex with others or just voyeurism (see page 139). This term has many definitions, depending on who is doing the defining, so make sure you know what the specific person means when using the term before you get naked with him or her.

* **SPLIT ROAST:** Generally describes a threesome in which one member is penetrated vaginally or anally by another while giving oral sex to the third but also may be used to describe the classic 69 position.
* **THREESOME:** Describes sex between a couple and another person; it might be two men and a woman, two women and a man, three men, or three women.
* **VOYEUR:** A person who watches others engage in sexual acts and does not join the action.

A threesome is sexual activity in which three people participate, generally a couple and another person. Fair enough, but that's not all there is to it, clearly. There are levels of involvement for each of the participants, and there are usually pretty clear rules about who's going to do what to whom, what isn't allowed, and how you'll let the other participants know if a boundary has been crossed. But the first step, before deciding any of this, is to decide if in fact you want to participate in a threesome.

Note: In this section, we are mainly addressing couples thinking about having a threesome. For single people who want to join a couple in a threesome, most of this advice still works, but a lot more talking and consensus needs to happen within a couple, so we are focusing there.

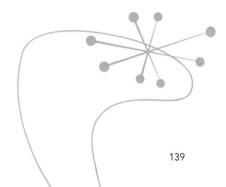

FOR COUPLES WHO ARE CONTEMPLATING ADDING A THIRD

Quiz #1

Are you and your partner ready for a threesome?

Read each of the statements below and check the ones that apply to your relationship:

❑ We are committed to each other and secure in our relationship.

❑ We are open about our sexual fantasies and share them with each other.

❑ One or both of us fantasizes about asking another person to join us in a sexual encounter.

❑ Neither of us is a jealous person.

❑ We can both separate our loving relationship from sex.

❑ Experimenting sexually is very important to both of us.

❑ One or both of us is bisexual or bicurious.

❑ Both of us would enjoy seeing our partner being pleased by someone else.

❑ If we try something new sexually and it's not great for one or both of us, we can get past it.

❑ We are both able to have sex without getting emotionally involved.

If you and your partner checked off the first five statements, you're receptive to the idea of a threesome. Each statement you checked off after the first five means you're one step closer to deciding to have one. If you checked off all ten, you're raring to go!

Quiz #2:

Who should not have a threesome?

Read each of the statements below and check the ones that apply to your relationship:

- ❏ One or both of us is concerned that we're just not wild enough in the bedroom.

- ❏ We are bored with our sex life and want to spice it up.

- ❏ One or both of us experienced a threesome before (with other partners) and wants to do it again.

- ❏ One or both of us is afraid we'll cheat on our partner and we think this is a solution.

- ❏ One or both of us has a jealous personality type.

- ❏ I want to test my significant other to see if he or she will cheat on me if given the chance.

- ❏ We have trouble communicating about what each of us wants out of our sex life.

- ❏ One of us thinks he or she might be gay/straight (depending on relationship orientation).

If you and your partner checked even one of these statements, you need to have about three years' worth of honest conversation before you even contemplate inviting another person into your bed.

BARE FACTS

The fact is, your relationship must be as strong as your desire to have a threesome before you should even discuss it. And you'd best discuss it fully clothed, too—not just as part of pillow talk.

A threesome is not a way to subvert two-timing tendencies or get your partner to open up about what he wants you to do to him when he's naked. It's probably true that lots of threesomes happen as a result of each of the reasons in the second quiz, and that's unfortunate, because it's not a good idea to take a relationship that's on shaky ground already and throw it into an earthquake. Make no mistake: a threesome will shake up your relationship no matter how much you've fantasized about it and discussed it and planned it and looked forward to it. It might be great, it might be all you hoped it would be, but things will be different in your relationship when it's over. That's why reality is so different from fantasy and why for couples a threesome should not be a spur-of-the-moment decision that is entered into lightly.

DON'T BE A JERK

The fact that your favorite twentieth-century psychoanalyst forced his wife to accept a third person into their relationship (and she put up with it for decades) doesn't mean it's ever okay to force or overly persuade your partner into a threesome. Things will not end well.

If you're sure you want to do it, read on and discover the who, what, when, where, and how of threesomes.

BEGINNING THE JOURNEY

You and your partner had a passionate sex session last night—it really got going when she mentioned how hot it would be if she could be having anal and vaginal sex at the same time. You got out the dildo and simulated it, and she had one amazing orgasm after another. It was pretty fantastic for you, too, and now, the next day, you're thinking about how incredible the fantasy was and how much you might like to try it out in real life. So . . . how do you broach the topic with your partner?

The good news is that because you are open and honest about fantasies, it won't be an enormous, ridiculous jump to discuss the possibility of a real live threesome.

SNAP OF THE FINGER

For those of you who don't talk about fantasies and are thinking of a threesome, start smaller. Try talking about toys or fantasies first so that you don't precipitate a coronary in the love of your life.

If you have a generally open and honest relationship already, bringing up the idea of a threesome shouldn't cause anyone to get upset or be shocked. It is, however, a matter to be handled delicately.

Assuming your initial statement (for example, "So, honey, how would you feel about maybe making that fantasy of two people pleasing you at once a reality?") isn't met with tears or hand-wringing, there are probably a lot of questions that will be asked, and you'll need to answer them honestly and with a fair amount of sensitivity. If your relationship is solid and healthy, that shouldn't be a problem.

COMMON INITIAL QUESTIONS

* Why do you want to do this? Aren't I enough for you?
* Are you gay or bisexual?
* Do you still love me?
* Is this just an excuse to do it with someone else?
* What about our wedding vows?
* Are you cheating on me?
* Will you leave me if I don't do this?
* If I do it, do I have to have sex with someone of my own gender?

If you bring it up and your partner has any of these questions, answer them honestly. If he or she is assuaged and receptive to the idea after you've done this, wonderful. If not, you may feel that you should try talking your partner into going through with a threesome. This is not a good idea. You both must want it; one partner should not just go along with it. That partner probably won't enjoy it, and that's a perfect recipe for resentment, from which no relationship benefits.

If the initial discussion did not go well, let the issue lie for a good long time. If after several months you are still interested in pursuing a threesome, try again. If not, it's no skin off your nose.

Or, if you're lucky, you're both on exactly the same page and really want to do it individually and as a couple, and all that's left is to work out the details before you're blissfully on your way to a soft-swinging situation. Good for you!

Once it's decided that you will do it, though, there are still questions to be asked and answered, and this is where you'll need to take a look at yourselves and your relationship and make sure a threesome is what you both want.

SECOND-STEP QUESTIONS

* What do we hope to get out of this experience?
* If it doesn't go well, will we be able to talk about it and move on?
* Will I be able to watch my partner having sex with another person?
* What would I like to happen during a threesome?
* What would I absolutely not like to happen during a threesome?
* How much work am I willing to do to make this happen for us?
* Will our relationship be strengthened and intensified if we do this?
* Will our relationship suffer if we do this?

Once you and your partner have really talked about these issues openly and honestly, you must again assess whether you want to have a threesome. If the answer is yes, there is *yet another* set of questions to go over together.

LISTEN UP, THIS IS IMPORTANT

It's probably a good idea to identify the gender of the third person in your proposed threesome early in the negotiations. Otherwise, the two of you may have very different ideas in your heads.

ADVANCED NEGOTIATIONS

1. Do we want a man or a woman to join us for a threesome?
2. Do we want to ask a stranger or someone we know?
3. How will we find someone without seeming creepy or weird?

4. Do we want to meet in our home or somewhere else?
5. What rules and boundaries must be set before the threesome experience?

Now let's break down how to answer these questions for your specific relationship and situation.

Whether you want your third to be a boy or a girl is a pretty important thing to decide, no? The answer depends on what each of you wishes to get out of the threesome experience. Everyone's situation is different, of course, but you can omit one sex or the other pretty easily:

* If you are a man and your female partner wants double penetration and doesn't want to share you with another woman and you are curious about what it might be like to suck dick, you probably want a gentleman to join you (though you might not want him to act like one!).
* If you are a straight woman who is bicurious and doesn't mind seeing your male partner in a sexual situation with another woman and your male partner has always wanted to see two women have sex, a woman as your third is probably a safe bet.
* Maybe you are in a same-sex relationship and would like to ask someone of the opposite sex to join you to see what it's like or for any other reason, or you'd like to ask another person of the same sex because voyeurism is your thing or to fully realize a fantasy.

Who to ask is a tough decision, especially if you decide to ask someone you know. This is a risky proposition, largely because in addition to changing the relationship between the two of you as a couple, your relationship with a third person with whom you are already friends with will also change. A lot. But still, lots of folks want to have a threesome specifically because both members of the couple are attracted to someone they both know. So if it's a friend you'd like to ask, be cautious and be aware that if he or she says no, your relationship will still change.

BARE FACTS

Even if you don't all get naked together, the fact that you asked your buddy to get naked with you and your partner could make fantasy football sessions or a book club a tad uncomfortable.

So perhaps you want to find a stranger, someone with whom it will definitely not be awkward with afterward, because you will never have to see that person again at the work Christmas party, say, or at the gym. This is perhaps the most personal choice of all when you're contemplating a threesome, and it's a decision the two of you will have to make together. Just remember to consider the consequences.

If you decide on a stranger, there are a number of avenues you might pursue to find a person to whom you are both attracted and who will be a welcome addition to your bed. The main ways to go about finding a third are these:

* *Lifestyle clubs.* These are basically swingers' clubs where couples and singles can go to check one another out and then all play together. Not all clubs allow sex, though, so make sure you know which kind you are in. The major bonus with these clubs is that your first introduction is face to face—you won't have to worry that the person won't show up. The drawback is that swingers' clubs do

not cater to threesomes specifically but to all kinds of group sex. Also, there isn't a lifestyle club on every corner, not even in these progressive times, so you might have to travel a bit to find one.

* *The mighty Internet.* There are so many adult dating sites online that it would be insane to try to list them here, but Adult FriendFinder (adultfriendfinder.com) and Adult Find Out (adultfindout.com) are popular and allow you to specify exactly what you want.

SECRET TIP

Many adult dating sites are free, which is a big plus since you're probably going to want to spend all your money on lube anyway.

* *If you want to keep it very local and you're in a fairly large metropolitan area, a good place to try is your city's alternative newsweekly's personals page.* These pages are generally chockablock with folks seeking all manner of kinky fun. The drawbacks with adult personal ads are the same as those with regular ones: People lie. The person you choose might not be "model beautiful" or have a "ten-inch love rod" or might not even show up. Also, someone might see you online—someone you don't want to know you're trolling the Internet for a third to visit your bedroom. And it may take some time to find someone, since there are tons of folks out there looking to spice it up. But you've already committed to spending quite a bit of time on this, so that shouldn't deter you.

* *Regular bars or clubs.* This is a less daunting option for sure, but the chances of finding someone whom you both find attractive *and* who is open to the idea are slim to none.

The decision on where to meet is based on several factors, though perhaps none is as important as your comfort level. If your third is a friend and lives near you, it probably wouldn't hurt to talk about it at your own place and then do it there, too. If your third is a person whom you're meeting specifically for a threesome, you might not be comfortable having the initial meeting in your home because the person is a stranger and you may feel that your bedroom is for you and your partner alone and that a threesome should happen outside it, in a hotel or vacation home or the like. There is also the issue of how far this person lives from you; if it's a good distance, you might not have a choice except to meet somewhere in the middle. For some people hoping to engage in a threesome, the money for a room might also be a concern.

Deciding on the rules and setting boundaries for the experience is maybe the most important preliminary step to having a threesome. This is where you'll figure out what you both want and don't want from the encounter, and you should hold nothing back at this stage. You need to be comfortable talking about how you want the threesome to go, or else how will you ever be comfortable enough to participate? This deserves its own section.

SETTING BOUNDARIES

Here are some rules that should jump-start a discussion of boundaries and make the threesome experience safe and enjoyable for all involved:

1. Be selective about who you invite into your bed!
2. Get comfortable with your body.
3. Be honest about your boundaries.
4. Don't do anything any of the participants is uncomfortable with.
5. Always use condoms and/or dental dams; unprotected sex is not an option.
6. Don't drink more than one or two alcoholic beverages to get loosened up; being drunk will compromise your ability to play it safe.
7. For your first threesome, don't perform any sex acts with the third person that you've never done with your partner.
8. Respect all participants' boundaries.
9. Don't do anything you don't want to do.
10. Don't assume anything; always ask.

Some of this is common sense and some of it is a little less intuitive, but regardless of how obvious you think a rule is, you should discuss it with your partner.

It's very important to decide on your personal level of involvement before you are actually naked with two people. For example, if you only want to watch your partner get it on with someone else, you need to let your partner know (and your third, but that comes later). If you're willing to perform oral sex on your third but don't want that person going down on you or if it's okay with you for your partner to perform oral sex but not penetrate the third with his penis, you need to tell your partner.

It might seem ridiculous to have to spell all this out, or it might seem like it doesn't leave room for spontaneity, and that's true: it doesn't.

YOU'RE WELCOME FOR THE TIP

Spontaneity seems like a great idea only until you're naked and uncomfortable and your partner is obliviously having sex with someone who is not you while you watch.

Another important boundary to set for mixed-sex threesomes (as opposed to same-sex ones) is how much same-sex contact you or your partner is comfortable with. You may be a woman who is way psyched to make out with another woman but doesn't want to be involved in a girl-on-girl cunnilingus situation. Or you're a man who's always wanted to go down on another guy but you're absolutely *not* okay with having anal intercourse with him. These specific parameters need to be itemized. If same-sex behavior makes you uncomfortable, having a "let the chips fall where they may" attitude will not serve you well during a threesome. This experience *is* supposed to be fun, after all. Setting clear boundaries will help ensure that it is all you hoped it would be.

Of course, if you and your partner discuss all this and decide that each of you really is okay with whatever might happen—and you've considered every permutation of sex that might happen—then by all means, let the chips fall where they may. Go wild!

MAKING IT HAPPEN

Once you've selected a third and set firm boundaries with your partner, it's time to arrange the initial meeting with the person with whom you'd like to have a threesome.

Some tips for setting up the first meeting:

* Be honest. As in every stage of this endeavor, honesty is key. What good will lying do, after all? You'll just end up in a situation you don't want to be in.
* Meet first in a public place. This helps ensure the physical and emotional safety of everyone involved. It also makes it easier to ditch your intended third if he or she isn't what you want upon closer inspection. It would be much harder to get that person to leave your home than to leave a bar or restaurant.
* Don't plan the actual threesome for the first meeting. Give yourself time to get to know the person, if it's not someone you already know, and time to be really certain you're ready to go for it. There's no rush, so why not take the pressure off?

If the first meeting goes well and you're ready to take the next step (the threesome itself—duh), arrange the next meeting. When you speak with your third participant to arrange the meeting, that's the time to make sure he or she is crystal clear on your rules and boundaries.

Tell your third:

* Safe sex will be practiced at all times.

* If at any time you or your partner is uncomfortable or does not want to continue for any reason, you can stop the encounter.

* No drugs are allowed.

* Another meeting is not a given; that's something you and your partner will decide once you've experienced this one and talked about it.

* Any specific things that are not to be done to or with you or your partner (from the boundaries you set already).

* A clean bill of health in the form of negative AIDS and sexually transmitted disease test results would be nice to see.

* Decide whether you will all spend the whole night together or if your guest will leave at a prearranged time.

TONIGHT'S THE NIGHT

By now you, your partner, and the third participant should be old pals, totally comfortable with one another, right? With any luck, you won't feel nervous or anxious when the big day arrives, but more likely than not and even if you've talked a blue streak with this person already, you'll be a little on edge.

First of all, a drink or two should provide the social lubrication and liquid courage you need to get relaxed and enjoy the fantasy that's being realized. But don't have more than that! If you're drunk, not only will you be less able to pay attention to what's going on and less in touch with your senses, but also, more important, you'll be less likely to be strict about playing it safe. So have a glass of wine or even two, but stop there.

While you sip your drink, try one of these icebreaking activities at the start of the encounter:

* Play strip poker or a naughty board game. Sex shops have a wide variety of suggestive games, and shopping for them will be a fun activity for you and your partner. You can even try a regular card game or board game if you want. It might take the pressure off to keep your clothes on for a while at the start of the adventure.

* Each one of you tells a funny sex story from your past. Remember the time you did it at the public pool after hours and got caught by your friend's dad, who was a cop? Or that time you gave your boyfriend a blowjob while you drove home for Christmas from college? Telling stories will enhance the camaraderie between a couple and a third; it will also make you laugh, which will relax you, too.

* Grab your digital camera or Polaroid and take some sexy pictures. You don't have to get completely naked, and you can be silly instead of sexy if you want. Vamping for the camera should get you loose either way.

* Dance. Start with fast music to get your adrenaline flowing, then slow it down and see what develops. Chances are that a sensual slow dance will get you right where you want to be.

* Read some erotica aloud. Pick a story from this book, maybe, and then see if the three of you can't create an erotic scenario of your own.

* Play truth or dare. Start tame, with mostly truth questions, and then move on to naughty dares. This should get your juices flowing—creative and otherwise!

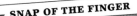

SNAP OF THE FINGER

When all else fails, try some porn. You might start out by making fun of it—the silly dialogue, the enormous fake breasts—but eventually it probably will have the desired effect. Then you can turn it off.

ESSENTIAL THREESOME ETIQUETTE

As far as positions go, who's doing what to whom at any given moment and who should climax first, second, and third, we wouldn't presume to tell you, and you probably can work out most of the configurations by taking into account everyone's desires and boundaries.

YOU'RE WELCOME FOR THE TIP

Positions during the real thing will be very different from what you were able to accomplish when it was just the two of you and a dildo. Dildos don't have arms and legs and heads, after all; this makes reality a bit more awkward and, of course, more real.

We can, however, offer are some suggestions and helpful hints so that you don't end up tangled in a heap or disappointed by what should be—if you've made it this far—a phenomenal sexual experience for all three of you.

* Don't use porn as a guideline. Take this advice to heart in two senses:

    1. Porno directors are in the business of making fantasy fodder that looks good. There are special lights and scene setters to make sure it looks good. You won't have those things, so it may not always look great or go smoothly. It may be difficult to figure out where to put your arm or leg sometimes. Try to go with the flow and don't worry too much about how it looks.

    2. Porn is not known for its loving relationships, but presumably, you and your partner are in one. Having a threesome does not mean you shouldn't be tender toward your partner and let him or her know that even though there's an exciting new person in your bed, you're still very much in love with your partner.

* Try to keep everyone involved at all times. Nothing makes a person feel more unwanted than being naked and left out of a threesome.

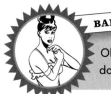

BARE FACTS

Obviously, if one person is there just to watch, you don't have to involve him or her in the sex.

* If something happens that you don't enjoy or that makes you feel uncomfortable, let it be known without unnecessarily hurting someone's feelings or spoiling the mood. In other words, try to be forthright and polite at the same time.

* As with any sexual situation, toys and accessories can be a welcome addition. They may include vibrators, lubricants (highly

recommended), blindfolds, or any other accoutrements you might enjoy. Just make sure everyone's on board.

✳ Each participant should take a turn being the center of attention. It's only fair that everyone be spoiled!

✳ It cannot be stressed enough: Condoms and dental dams are a must!

✳ Take your time. This might be a once-in-a-lifetime experience, and so it should be savored. And if it's not just a one-off, then why try to do everything the first time? Don't rush. It'll be much better if you take it slow and enjoy yourself.

✳ Pay attention to your partner. Sexually, of course, but also pay attention to what he or she seems to be enjoying with your guest. If part of the reason you decided to have a threesome was to gain a deeper understanding of your partner's sexuality and your own, firsthand knowledge is best. It's right there for you to see, so take a good long look.

QUICK FIX

There will inevitably be some downtime during the threesome. Each participant may find him or herself without something (or someone) to do for a few minutes. Take this time to masturbate or enjoy the show—or hey, do both!

WHAT HAPPENS NEXT?

Sometime after your experience (though probably not immediately after your guest departs, as you will probably be kind of sleepy), you and your partner need to discuss the encounter.

That's right: more questions.

* Did each of you get what you wanted out of it?

* Did it meet your expectations?

* Did you enjoy yourself?

* Did any part of it make you feel uncomfortable or bad?

* What feelings, besides arousal, did you experience during the encounter?

* If you were to do it again, are there things you would do differently?

* Do you want to do it again?

* If the two of you do it again, would you invite the same third person back?

* What did you learn about your own sexual identity?

* What did you learn about your partner's sexuality?

These questions will help you decide whether you want to make threesomes a regular part of your sexual repertoire or if once was enough to satisfy your urge and curiosity. Your feelings about the experience may change, so keep talking about it as that happens. If nothing else comes of your threesome experience, you will have learned to talk openly about sexual matters with your partner, and that is an extremely important skill. If you decide to do it again, have a blast!

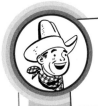

WELL, LOOK WHO FINALLY MADE THE *Rodeo*

For something that sounds so **RISKY**, inviting a third person to share your bed involves **RESEARCH, CAREFUL QUESTIONS,** and **HONEST ANSWERS**, and an awareness that no matter what happens, even simply bringing the subject up can change a relationship for better or worse. We hope it's for the better!

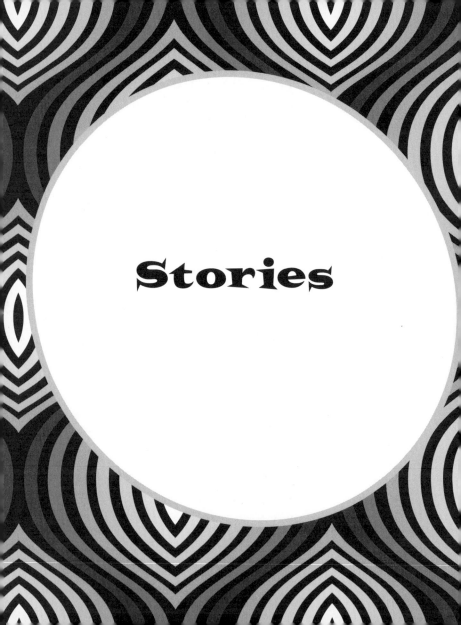

Stories

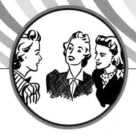

LONG WEEKEND

Anne Alexander

"Oh, yes," Tricia purred, sinking deeper into the steamy water. "This is just what I needed."

"Mmmm, me too," Julie said, lifting one of her long, toned legs out of the Jacuzzi and wiggling her toes.

"Yeah, this was a great idea. I'm so glad I had it!" Lindy laughed, thinking of that day two months ago when she'd e-mailed her two best friends from college with a plan: they would all meet in Vegas for a long weekend, stay somewhere fancy, and really have a wild time together, the way they used to. It had been too long since they'd all been together, probably since her brother's wedding the previous year. Even though they were all busy with their separate lives in their different cities, they'd stayed very close in the ten years since graduating. But it had definitely been too long this time.

And now here they all were, in a hot tub in a deluxe suite at the Bellagio, looking out over the Las Vegas strip while immersed in hot, swirling water. They'd arrived the night before and gone right out to dinner, then to a club, then to the casino, and then finally back to the suite, where they'd fallen into bed around 4 a.m. They were taking it easy today, just relaxing, since each had been stressed at work lately and they all really needed some downtime. After shopping and walking around town all day, the Jacuzzi proved the perfect thing.

Julie sipped her champagne and then said, "So, do you think we'll meet any guys tonight? They were all duds last night."

"Ugh, who cares? I don't want to think about it," Lindy said. "We came here to get *away* from stress, right?"

"True. And anyway, I think Gary would be a little peeved if I hooked up on this vacation," Tricia said.

"I thought you guys were off again. What's up?" Lindy asked.

"Oh, I don't know. I can't keep up. I don't even want to talk about it. Turn up the jets?" Tricia sighed.

"You got it." Julie reached over and turned the knob.

They sat in relaxed silence for a few minutes, luxuriating in the water bubbling around their bodies. Then Tricia sat up, grabbed her glass, and asked, "Anyone need more champers? I'm thirsty!"

"I'll take some more, though I'm feeling a little tipsy," Julie said, handing over her glass.

"Me, too," Lindy said, her voice thick with happy, sleepy relaxation.

Tricia stood up in a whoosh, and the water splashed down her naked body, forming droplets on the ends of her nipples, which had hardened from the cool air outside the tub. Her dark hair was wisped around her face, and she was all pink from the hot water. Lindy looked up at her. "You look beautiful, Trish," she said.

"Aw, thanks, babe. You're not too bad yourself." Tricia winked, scampered out of the tub, and headed for the bar. She returned in a moment with the champagne bottle, setting it on the edge of the Jacuzzi and climbing back in.

Julie reached out her glass, giggling. "Fill me up!" she said.

When everyone had a full glass again, Lindy said, "A toast!" They all raised their glasses. "To staying best friends and staying close. I love you guys."

"Aw, I love you guys," Tricia said, leaning over and kissing Lindy on the cheek.

"I love you, too!" Julie said, turning her head to kiss Tricia just as Tricia turned her head. They ended up colliding and kissing on the lips. They were moving a bit slowly because of all the bubbly, and they held the kiss for a moment.

"Oooooh," Lindy said. Then, "Hey! No fair! I want a kiss." Julie broke from Tricia and leaned over to Lindy.

"Aw, you feel left out, Lin? I'll kiss you," she teased, planting a soft kiss on her friend's lips.

"I will, too!" Tricia shouted, leaning over and kissing Lindy on the cheek, then moving to her mouth as Julie drew back and took a sip from her glass.

"You guys?" Julie said tentatively. "I just had an idea. In the spirit of, you know, relaxation and girl power and how much we all love each other—"

"Oh, shut up, Julie," Tricia said, putting her mouth over her friend's to make her quiet. Tricia reached her hand up and took the clip out of her friend's curly blond hair, letting it fall around her face. "This what you had in mind?"

Julie nodded as Lindy reached her hand down to feel Tricia's breast, gently tweaking the nipple she had admired a few minutes before. In response, Tricia reached her own hand back and flicked Lindy's pink-tipped breast with her fingers. She broke the kiss with Julie just long enough to say, "Lindy, I've always loved your boobs. They're so great."

Lindy blushed, moved her wet black locks out of the way, and looked down at her breasts. They were pretty nice even though she'd often wished her double-Ds were a little smaller. "Thanks, Trish. I like yours, too," she said, dripping some champagne down onto Tricia's chest and then bending down to lick the sweet liquid from her friend's perky breast.

Julie reached over and turned the jets down. "What about mine, you guys?" she said, sticking them out.

Tricia and Lindy laughed as each reached out a hand to finger one of Julie's gorgeous silver-dollar-sized beauties. "Perfect," Tricia sighed.

"Really wonderful, Jules," Lindy said, leaning in to kiss Julie. Julie's lips parted immediately, and Lindy took the opportunity to push her tongue into her friend's luscious mouth. Soon their tongues were wrestling feverishly as they toyed with each other's hard nipples.

"Wow, you guys are so lovely," Tricia said.

Lindy and Julie broke their kiss, giggling. "I think she's drunk," Lindy said.

"I am, but you're still lovely," Tricia said, pouting. "Now one of you, come sit on my lap."

Julie hopped up, water cascading down her petite figure, and straddled Tricia, facing out toward Lindy. Tricia pulled Julie's hair to the side and immediately began kissing and nibbling her neck, eliciting a delighted moan from her. Lindy covered Julie's mouth with her own once again, and the two women began a slow, deep kiss.

After a few rapturous moments of this, Lindy reached her hand down under the water toward the spot between Julie's legs that she knew must be on fire, only to find Tricia's hand already there. She was momentarily disappointed but then decided Tricia probably needed attention, too, and reached her hand past Julie's tight, round ass into the slippery spot between Tricia's legs.

"Ohhh," Tricia moaned against Julie's neck as Lindy's fingers plunged inside her first tentatively and then with more force.

Lindy could tell from her friend's whimpers that Tricia was enjoying her ministrations. (And why not? Lindy thought, I always enjoy myself when I masturbate!) But Lindy was feeling neglected even though Julie was playing with her nipples nonstop. Her clitoris was aching for some attention, though, and she just had to have it, so she maneuvered herself up onto her knees and scooted her butt backward, finding a pulsing jet. She positioned her clit over the jet and sank down a little to get a better fit.

"Mmmm, yeah," she said as Julie's hand, which had momentarily lost Lindy's nipple when she shifted her position, found the stiff bud once more. Meanwhile, Tricia was rubbing right above Julie's clit, where she knew her friend loved to be stroked.

Back in college, there wasn't much the three friends didn't share with one another, and how they masturbated and the specifics of their sexual encounters were well-covered topics among them. Each knew how the others came hardest and best, and each was intent on pleasing her friends.

Lindy's new position didn't allow her access to Tricia, so she sat back down, suddenly missing the jet's position on her clitoris. Her hand quickly found Tricia's again, and she tickled it lightly and then dipped inside her friend again. With her other hand, Lindy grabbed Julie's free hand and placed it on her own sweet spot. Julie's eyes opened as she was momentarily taken out of her reverie, but she quickly got the message and began stroking Lindy in earnest, pausing every once in a while to stick two fingers inside her and lean down and lightly bite a nipple.

One of Tricia's hands had moved to Julie's breasts, and between that attention and the hand that had been steadily moving between her legs, Julie was nearly at her peak. The sensations her friends were giving her and the pulsating hot water all around her got to be too much as she suddenly felt herself coming. "Oh, you guys, oh! Jesus. Mm, oh," she babbled incoherently as her vaginal walls tightened around Tricia's fingers and her belly shook through her climax.

"Ahh," she breathed, catching her breath.

"No rest for the wicked!" Lindy teased, finding Julie's lips with her own yet again. Feeling how breathless Julie was as she pushed her tongue into her mouth, Lindy felt herself going over the edge in just a moment as Julie's fingers moved right down onto her clitoris and increased the pressure. Lindy murmured into Julie's mouth as she lost her grip on reality, slowly letting herself fall over the cliff of pleasure. "Right there, right there, yes!" she exclaimed as she went perfectly still and came. Hard. For several moments.

As Lindy came down, Tricia cleared her throat. Julie and Lindy both giggled and turned their attention to Tricia. Julie leaned down and took a hard nipple into her mouth as Lindy's hands found what they were looking for: One lightly teased Tricia's clitoris as the other traced around her vagina and then moved inside it. Lindy leaned over and kissed Tricia's earlobe then, gently licking the soft flesh and then blowing ever so softly on it. That was it; that was all Tricia needed, and Lindy had known it.

"Oh damn, yes! Yes! Yes! I'm there, I'm there, yes!" she yelled, and then she collapsed into her friends, giggling.

"Oh, gosh, that's right; she said she always cracks up after she comes," Lindy noted, giggling herself.

Julie joined in, too. "I guess we know each other pretty well, huh?"

"I guess so," Tricia said, still panting.

"I guess we didn't need to meet any guys tonight, right?" Julie said, recalling their earlier conversation.

They all looked at one another, then burst out laughing again.

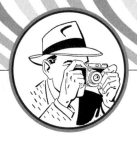

PHOTO FINISH

C. M. Bradley

I've been a professional photographer and owner of my own studio for just over ten years. To attract new business, I began what is called boudoir photography. For those of you who aren't aware of what that involves, it usually consists of a curious woman who wants to take revealing portraits of herself for a significant other. I wasn't aware of how many people in my area would be interested in this type of photograph. During the sessions, I had a few customers ask if I did videos as well. Initially, the answer was no. However, after numerous requests, I expanded my craft to include boudoir videos. I found that most people wanted that kind of work done within their homes, so I had to expand with the times and take my work on the road.

I received a request for boudoir photographs from Ms. Sandra H. She's an outgoing young woman who works as a store manager in the local Super Store. Upon arriving at her home, which she shares with Mark, her fiancé, I received a warm greeting. She insisted that I call her Sandy. Sandy and I sat in her airy kitchen, where she prepared some coffee and began explaining that the photographs were an anniversary gift. Sandy had specific ideas and poses. She thought she should run them past me before we started. Her ideas were a little unusual and definitely fell within the realm of the erotic. However, I agreed, and she escorted me into the bedroom so that I could set up my equipment.

Sandy entered the room wearing a robe and carrying adult toys. She arranged the bed, and I discreetly arranged the lighting equipment along with the crotch of my pants. I suggested a few practice shots with her robe on to give us both a chance to get comfortable with the setting. Even before she removed her robe, I could see that she was more endowed than I had suspected. After approximately twenty minutes, we took a break and chatted. That was when Sandy openly revealed that she wanted some of the photos to appear as if she were having intercourse with another man. Sandy confided in me that it was her fiancé's fantasy to see her having sex with another man. She didn't mind his fantasy because she secretly desired it as well, only her profession and personality didn't afford her the opportunity to act on that fantasy. She related that she trusted me because of my reputation and had thus far been very satisfied with my level of service.

After our brief respite, we returned to the makeshift photo studio and began the actual session. Gradually, Sandy opened her robe, revealing her smooth, milky skin. She was shy at first but warmed up to the camera and me like a pro. After several teasing poses were completed, the poses became more graphic. Nipples and pubic hair became visible with each feminine pose. Hand placement became critical and most arousing. I knew she saw the erection I was sporting in my loose-fitting trousers, but I maintained a professional demeanor. After a sufficient selection of shots had been taken, Sandy broke out an "ethnic" dildo. The dildo was as dark as me but put me to shame in length and girth.

Sandy appeared uncomfortable as she explained, "In my fantasies, I am being penetrated by my Mandingo." She blushed as she felt the need to apologize again and again.

I just replied with, "Sandy, it was toys like that one that kept me in demand during my college years."

My humorous response brought a smile to her face and visible relaxation to her voluptuous body. It had been determined that my shots would not reveal that the adult toy was just a prop. The photos would have to show her face and appear as though a man, a black man, were pleasuring her.

The shots included oral, which was not a problem. The rear entry shots were a little trickier. I must admit that some of my repositioning of the prop while it was protruding from her orifice might have been unnecessary. But I think we both enjoyed the hell out of it. Our final poses consisted of her lying on her back and fully inserting the prop into her now obviously juicy center. I did the best I could to achieve the objective, but from the sensuous, preoccupied look on her face I didn't think it mattered.

We collected ourselves and proceeded into the living room, where I arranged a viewing of our digital endeavor. Sandy sat on the couch with a fresh cup of coffee, wearing only her robe, and crossed her legs. The view of her leg through her partially opened robe was breathtaking. I had suddenly become a leg man. I stood next to the screen like an instructor teaching a captivated classroom of students. As each photo appeared on the large plasma screen, one more erotic than the next, I could tell she was pleased with what she was viewing. The look on her face and the way she recrossed her legs indicated that something was going on in her nether region. We discussed a possible future project involving video as she wrote a check. Sandy expected that Mark would love the photos and acquiesce to her request for a video. We exchanged eye contact and mischievous smirks as I departed from her home.

A week later, Sandy contacted me, relating that Mark had indeed loved the photos. According to Sandy, the only problem Mark would have had with the session was that if in fact someone was having sex with her, he would have wanted to be there. It seemed to me that Sandy expressed that statement with a hint of glee in her voice. Sandy also related that Mark had agreed to participate in her proposed video project. Sandy and I then scheduled an appointment that Mark could attend. I agreed to meet them at their house so that we could get started immediately once the terms were set.

I arrived and was greeted by Mark. We shook hands, and he immediately began praising my work. I was escorted into the living room, where Sandy was enjoying a drink. Mark offered me a refreshment while he prepared one for himself. I graciously declined and prepared to get down to business. Mark then ran the photo session as a slide show on their large television. Each erotic shot of his lovely Sandy was clicking across the screen while we discussed his critique of the poses. Mark took great care in describing the graphic situations he wanted me to capture. His primary concern was capturing Sandy giving him oral pleasure. Displaying the previous shots and discussing them with me was an effective way of making me aware that he was comfortable with the proposed graphic scenes. Sandy appeared pensive, almost as if she were scheming at the opposite end of the room. It wasn't until later that I discovered what Sandy had in mind. She was allowing Mark and me to get better acquainted before she put her plan into action.

Upon the completion of our discussion, everyone was clear on the graphic nature of the anticipated video. The terms were agreed on, and Mark left the room. Sandy remained behind allegedly to escort me to the bedroom with my equipment.

Sandy used that opportunity to say, "I would consider it a tremendous favor if you would participate in the action once the video is completed."

I didn't quite know how to respond. Sandy then reminded me, "It's Mark's fantasy to watch me having sex with another man." Sandy also said, "When the time is right, I'll give you a signal."

I just mumbled, "We'll see."

Sandy and Mark returned, wearing their appropriate attire, and waited for me to give them their cue. Once again, we took a practice run through a few positions so that we could all get comfortable. After a short break in which the final details were discussed, I prepared the camera and gave them the signal.

The erotic vignette began with Mark entering the bedroom wearing his bathrobe. Sandy was sitting on the bed in her negligee reading a book. He began kissing her on her ankles and working his way up her inner thighs. He then forcefully stretched her out onto the bed, opened her gown to reveal her breasts, and plunged his face between her legs. Once a close-up of the oral gratification was captured, he kissed way up her body to her nipples. I moved back for a wider angle to capture his stiffening member dangling out of his robe and trailing up her leg. Close-ups of Mark sucking and licking Sandy's nipples looked excellent through the camera's viewfinder. As planned, Mark then moved up and gave Sandy some passionate kisses.

After a few moments, Sandy took charge and pushed Mark onto his back. I was able to position myself just in time to film her straddling Mark and adjusting his member until it was nestled neatly in the crack of her ass. That view was obscured when Mark reached up and gently slid her sheer gown off her shoulders, allowing it to fall onto his legs. As he massaged her breasts, it was obvious that true emotion was flowing between them. Sandy leaned down and gave Mark a deep kiss. Her kisses and probing tongue moved slowly down his torso, stopping at his stiff cock. Sandy began working her magic on him. She had definitely perfected the art of fellatio. I now knew why Mark wanted to make sure Sandy's mastery of oral sex skills was captured on film. I could watch that for years to come myself.

Sandy's saliva coated Mark's genitals, which were devoid of hair. At that point it was obvious that Mark had temporarily taken up residence on cloud nine.

Sandy then used her index finger to beckon me to join the action and pointed to her ass, which was raised in the air. Initially I was hesitant, but I mentally referred to our discussions during the planning phase. I placed the camera on the tripod and removed only my pants. I positioned myself behind Sandy and pulled my throbbing tool and testicle sack through the slit of my boxers. My stiff dick easily slipped between the folds of skin as a result of the ample amount of natural lubrication supplied by Sandy. I watched my cock slowly disappear inside her. I could feel every ridge of her tight love canal as I entered. Once I obtained full penetration, my rhythm quickened. I held on to her waist and gave her full and steady thrusts. With each stroke, her juice matted my pubic hairs and dampened my boxers.

I was nearing my peak when the sound of my body slapping against Sandy's ass and Mark reaching his peak distracted me. I slowed my pace, opened my eyes, and observed Mark's body tensing up. Sandy began rolling Mark's cock across her cheek and lips. She was lovingly controlling the expulsion of his ejaculate onto her face. It was at that moment that I realized the difference between making love and having sex. Despite the sensations in my loins, I was doing the latter and felt like I was intruding. I quickened my pace so as not to fall too far behind Mark's completion. I completed a few more full strokes within that tight, wet pulsating canal and erupted. I released my firm grasp on Sandy's waist, watched my dick slowly regress from her moist crevice, and stepped back to catch my breath. I then observed my liquid release leaking down Sandy's thigh. Yes, I admit that I was quite pleased with myself.

As Mark was rising from the bed, I returned my manhood to my boxers and began gathering my equipment. Mark proceeded to the bathroom without a word. Sandy sighed and stretched out on the bed.

She interrupted my packing by asking me to come over to the bed. I stepped closer and she stated, "I wanna taste it."

Before the gears in the big head could turn, Sandy reached into my boxers and pulled out the little head. I felt my flaccid penis sliding past her wet lips and touching the back of her throat.

The subsequent growth was stunted by Mark's return. Mark paused and appeared to visually scan Sandy's body from the tip of her toes to her mouth, which was currently engulfing my penis. Mark opened his robe and started massaging his cock until it was fully erect. I remained frozen in time and space. I was unable to achieve a full erection and unable to turn away. As if watching a porno film, I stood there watching until Mark yanked his load across Sandy's ass and back. Mark had pleasured himself to exhaustion and fell across the bed. Sandy allowed my cock to slip out of her mouth and rolled toward Mark. In the midst of their cuddling, I determined that an immediate exit stage right was in order for me. I grabbed my pants and equipment and headed for the door.

As I exited the room, Sandy eased off the bed and grabbed her gown. I slipped on my pants as she put on her gown and moved toward me. Sandy whispered, "Thank you," and reminded me about my fee.

I found myself strangely aroused by the pungent aroma of sex emanating from Sandy and her shapely figure through that sheer gown, which was daintily being held closed by one hand. I related that she could drop off the check at my studio after they viewed the project. After all, if they didn't pay, I wouldn't have exactly felt cheated or wanted to explain that transaction in small claims court. I also said that if they weren't satisfied with the video, I would gladly schedule a retake. There were those mischievous smirks again as I left and scurried for the sanctuary of my car.

Although I never did business with Sandy again, I was promptly paid in full and had many referrals as a result of our pleasant encounter.

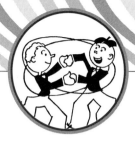

Spring Break

J. M. Thompson

John sat at the table, slowly sipping his iced tea and watching people walk by the window. He was waiting, hoping to see Joe show up. He wasn't sure if he would show—he hadn't been able to talk to him directly. Instead, he had left a message on his voice mail basically telling him he was in town for a day or so and would like to get together.

In high school and at the start of college, John had had two best friends, Joe and Mike. The three of them were rarely apart. They were the original Three Musketeers and the Three Stooges all rolled into an odd trio. They had finished high school together and headed out to the same university in Montgomery, Alabama. They remained great friends though the first year of college, and although Joe dropped out of school after that, they still hung out together as Mike and John worked through the second year at school. It was during spring break that year that their relationship changed.

Lifting his glass and nodding his head to the waitress, John got his tea refilled. He tore open a packet of sweetener and poured it into the tea and then took a sip as he remembered how excited the three friends were when they started out on that spring break. They were nearly three-quarters of the way to Pensacola Beach when they finally stopped for lunch.

John and Mike sat at the table betting on whether Joe would make it back from the jukebox before being accosted by some of the girls there. Joe was the complete ladies' man with long, straight dark hair that was always perfectly combed and deep dark brown eyes fringed with long eyelashes. He was thin, with features so delicate that he was usually more beautiful than any of the girls who chased him.

Sure enough, Joe suddenly veered off and sat down with a bunch of girls. Eventually, he would return to his friends' table with three of the girls, so Mike and John just sat and waited. Mike usually did well enough with the girls. He was a gymnast with blond hair and perfectly sculpted muscles. He didn't have the delicate features Joe did; he had a more rugged look, a distinctive nose, and a square cut to his jaw. He also was comfortable talking with pretty much anyone, and within minutes he could have even the most reticent person laughing out loud. Mike was definitely the clown of the three.

John was the slow one with the ladies. He was a football player in high school but wasn't good enough for college ball, and the lack of vigorous exercise at practice caused him to put on some pounds. He wasn't fat but was heavier than he felt comfortable about. This and his shyness were always problems for him when he met women.

Redirecting his thoughts back to that spring break, John remembered that it was Rod Stewart's "Maggie May" playing on the jukebox as Joe appeared at the table and invited the three girls to sit with them. For the next hour or so, Joe had the girls drooling, Mike kept the group laughing, and John sat quietly, worrying that they might not find a hotel with a room available if they didn't get moving. In the end, it turned out the girls were still in high school, and although Joe and Mike got their phone numbers, they tossed them once they got back in the car.

"Definite jailbait," Joe complained, starting his car.

"Hopefully the girls we meet at the beach will be in college," Mike replied.

"In college and ready to party," Joe said, flooring the car and speeding out toward the highway while the Guess Who blared on the cassette player, "*No sugar tonight for coffee. . . .*"

They arrived late at night but fortunately found a hotel with some vacancies, something that surprised John considering it was spring break. The three of them unloaded Joe's Plymouth Barracuda and stocked the room. It was after midnight when they finally crashed, Joe and Mike in the beds and John on the couch.

The next day they found the beach empty. They headed to a local restaurant for breakfast, where they learned that spring break for most of the local schools was not until the following week. That explained how they were able to get the room. They tried to make the best of it, swimming out into the ocean even though it was almost unbearably cold. While on the beach, Mike and Joe actually found a couple of local girls to hit on, but they had to head back to the mainland early in the afternoon. The three guys drank a few beers in the room before going to sleep that night.

Glancing at his watch, John thought that if Joe had gotten his message, he should be walking through the door of the restaurant in just a few minutes. He wondered if Joe still made the dramatic entries he always used to. John could see it now, that Barracuda pulling up to a space, Joe stepping out of the driver's seat, checking his hair in the side mirror, and then stepping into the room like he was some rock god.

Letting his mind slip back to the hotel room on the third night of their spring break trip, John remembered Joe barging into the bathroom with the same confident air with which he had entered every door John had seen. John was in the shower stroking himself slowly. As Joe pulled back the shower curtain, all John could do was stand there as the water slowly rinsed the soap off his erect cock. Joe simply reached out and gently grabbed it, moving his hand back and forth along the shaft.

"Turn off the water; I don't want to mess up my hair," John remembered Joe saying.

John reached over, turned off the water, and watched as Joe slowly knelt down. He gently pulled John's cock as he leaned forward. John watched in silence as Joe slid his mouth over his erection and began moving his head back and forth. John had been close to coming before Joe walked in, so it didn't take too long before he was breathing hard, pumping his hips back and forth.

Looking down, John saw his cock slipping in and out of the mouth of his friend. He moved his hands down and ran his fingers through Joe's hair, letting the sensations in his cock run through his entire body. Feeling the pleasure overtake him, he arched his back and came, spurting his cum into Joe's mouth. Without letting the cock slip from his mouth, Joe swallowed and continued sucking lightly as John's erection subsided.

Joe finally pulled away and gently milked the last drops of cum from John's cock. Joe licked up the last of it and then stood up, saying, "You better not have messed up my hair."

John grabbed a towel and quickly dried off as Joe stepped over to the sink and checked his hair in the mirror. He then slipped out of the bathroom. By the time John finished drying off, Joe was already naked, sitting on the edge of one of the beds. John looked between Joe's legs at his cock, seeing it erect for the first time. It was thin but quite a bit longer than John would have expected.

Joe slid backward on the bed and leaned back on the pillows as John crawled onto the bed and moved between his legs. He reached out and gently stroked his friend, watching as the pre-cum pooled in the tiny hole. Sticking out his tongue, John touched it to the tip of the cock and licked up the clear fluid. Surprised a bit at the bitter taste, he quickly moved his head forward, opened his mouth, and then closed it over Joe's cock.

As Joe moaned, John began sucking on the head of the cock as he continued stroking the shaft with his fingers. He tried to take as much of his friend's erection into his mouth as he could. He caught himself gagging a bit a couple of times as Joe thrust himself upward just as John moved his mouth down, but he quickly got into a rhythm where he didn't take too much into his mouth, and soon it felt just right.

Just as Joe really began to respond, they heard a key slide into the door. The door swung open, and Mike stepped in, saying, "Well I got the beer—What the hell?"

Still holding Joe's cock in his hand, John pulled his head back and looked up at Mike, not sure what to say. He glanced at Joe's face, but Joe remained silent too as he looked at Mike in what appeared to be sheer bewilderment. John looked back at Mike, opened his mouth, and then closed it. How could he explain it? Joe had barged in and then, well . . . something just happened.

John watched as Mike eyes slowly moved over them, starting with Joe's cock, which was still glistening with saliva, and then moving up Joe's body, finally staring right at his face. Mike's face reddened, and as John glanced down, he could see Mike's cock beginning to strain against his pants. Then, as if something inside him had snapped, Mike put the beer on the chair and began pulling off his shirt as if it were a completely natural thing to do.

Watching Mike continue to undress, John wondered what it was that had so suddenly taken them from best friends to this. Was it something they simply had felt all along, something they all longed for as they clowned around, or was it something more? Before he could think about it any more, he saw that Mike had removed his clothes and was moving toward them.

John immediately returned his attention to Joe's cock as Mike climbed onto the bed and crawled up near Joe's head. Pausing for a moment, he looked down as John continued sucking Joe's cock, his hand pumping up and down its long shaft. John then watched Mike lean forward as Joe turned his head and took Mike's cock into his mouth.

Not entirely confident in what he was doing, John watched what Joe did to Mike and basically did the same thing to Joe. Sure enough, in just a few minutes he could feel an urgency in Joe as he lifted his hips and tried to thrust his cock deeper into John's mouth. John responded by stroking Joe's shaft faster and sucking the head harder, running his tongue over it again and again. He was quickly rewarded—he saw Joe move his mouth from Mike's cock as he moaned loudly and came.

The warm spurts of cum caught John by surprise, and he tried to swallow the thick liquid without spilling any, but by the time Joe's orgasm had subsided, John had some of the white fluid running down his chin. He rested his head on Joe's thigh and watched as Joe returned his attention to Mike's cock, slurping hungrily on it. After a few minutes, Mike suddenly pushed his hips forward and came as Joe swallowed it all without spilling a drop. Only then did John stand up, walk over to the sink, and wipe off his face.

John broke from his reverie and glanced at his watch. Joe was fifteen minutes late now, and he began to think he might not show. "Maybe he just didn't get my message," he whispered, trying to convince himself there wasn't another reason for Joe not coming to see him. Looking back, he knew that wasn't true.

It wasn't until after three o'clock in the morning before the three lovers finally fell asleep, all entwined in one another's bodies on the bed. John woke up about nine the next morning and saw that both Joe and Mike were already gone. He got up, got dressed, and headed out to the beach, where he saw both of them sitting on some lounge chairs not far from the water.

John walked up and said, "Good morning," running his fingers through Joe's hair.

Joe jerked his head away and said angrily, "Hey, watch the hair. Now I'll have to wash it."

Figuring Joe was just sleep-deprived and grumpy, John sat down next to Mike, feeling his leg slightly rub against his friend's. Mike immediately jumped up and ran into the water, diving into a wave and swimming until he was about chest deep. John didn't think anything else about it until he learned that Mike and Joe had decided to check out of the hotel and head back home that day.

Well, they did miss the spring break rush and the skies were looking a bit cloudy, so John went along and packed up the car. The ride back to Montgomery was very quiet, with Mike sleeping most of the way and Joe driving in silence. Any conversation John tried to initiate was quickly rebuffed with Joe's short replies.

When they finally reached the school and John unloaded his stuff, he had to ask, "Guys, what is going on here?"

"What do you mean? Nothing's going on."

"But something happened, something very important. . . ." John started to say.

"Nothing happened, John, nothing at all," Joe replied.

"Something happened to me, we . . ."

"Don't pull Mike and me into this thing. Maybe something happened to you, it would happen to you, but nothing—understand me, nothing happened to us," Joe said, pointing at Mike and himself.

"But—"

"Look, I've always thought you were strange around girls; now I know why," Mike interrupted.

"But it was Joe—"

"It was nothing!" Joe shouted, climbing into his car.

John tried to say something more, but Joe started the car and was revving the engine. John just stood and watched as the car backed out and then sped away, the tires squealing and smoking as he left. That was the last time he talked to his friends.

In the fifteen or so years that followed, John learned that both did go on to get married and lead regular lives. Mike moved up north, and Joe pretty much stayed in Montgomery. Now John, on a business trip in Montgomery, glanced at his watch and saw that it was thirty-five minutes past the time he had asked Joe to meet him. He pulled out his wallet and paid the check.

Just as he was standing up from the table, he noticed the glass entry door to the restaurant swing open, and in stepped a tall, thin man with short but nicely groomed hair. His hair was dark with some distinguished graying along the temples. John watched as the man spotted a mirror and checked himself out before looking over the restaurant.

"John," he called out, waving.

John stepped forward and held out his hand, "Hi, Joe. I was afraid I might not recognize you."

"Yeah, it's the hair. I've been wearing it short lately. My wife says it makes me look dignified."

"Your hair is great as usual," John said as they moved to the table and sat down.

"It's been a long time, John," Joe said.

"Too long, Joe; it's been too long."

Joe looked at John and nodded. "Yes, too long."

HAPPY ANNIVERSARY!

Anne Alexander

Sure, I'm pretty uninhibited when it's just Tony and me, but boy was I nervous last month. It was our anniversary, and we had something really special planned. Something for just the two of us . . . and Jenny.

First of all, I guess I should say we'd both fantasized about having a woman join us in bed sometime—we'd talked about it during sex for years and even started researching it once or twice, only to get cold feet and call it quits at the last minute. We'd even set up a meeting once and then chickened out and canceled. But this time we were really ready, and there was no turning back.

It was our fifteenth wedding anniversary. Some people might think a threesome isn't a respectable or romantic way to celebrate that great accomplishment, but Tony and I thought realizing our biggest fantasy was the best way we could think of to commemorate such an event.

We met Jenny at a swingers' club, one of the ones where there's no actual sex in the club, just people trying to get acquainted to find someone they like. We were all nervous, but Jenny was cute and smart and sweet, with a great body. Tony and I were definitely both hot for her.

I guess I ought to mention I hadn't been with a woman since experimenting a little bit in college, but the idea had always turned me on, and it was something I wanted to explore further. And Tony—well, he's a man, so of course the idea of seeing two chicks getting it on excited him plenty. He was just a little skeptical at first, knowing as he did my predilection for checking out cute redheads, and was worried that maybe I'd grown tired of him or of men in general. But that wasn't it, and once he understood that, he was fully on board.

Jenny is, of course, redheaded, with blue eyes and gorgeous freckles. (I wouldn't find out till later—to my delight—that they were all over her body.) She's got a slightly larger frame than I do, taller and with bigger breasts. I'm sort of petite, with dark blond hair and small breasts. Tony always says I make up for that by having a great curvy ass. Such a sweetheart, my hubby. He's tall, over six feet, with dark hair. He's softened up a little in the middle over the years, but he's still a very sexy, good-looking guy. We're both in our late thirties, and Jenny just turned thirty.

Anyway, we all got along great at the club, had a few drinks, and talked for hours. We really got to know each other and laughed a lot. It went so well that we decided to set up the actual play date the weekend of our anniversary. We booked a suite at a fancy hotel just outside of our town. Then we waited with incredible anticipation—and some apprehension, too—for the weekend to come.

Eventually it arrived, and Tony and I got to the hotel first, checked in, and headed up to our suite. We opened the door and found ourselves in the lap of luxury.

The sitting room area was gorgeous, with a deep burgundy carpet and lighter rose-colored drapes. There were a couple of luxurious oversize sofas and natural wood end tables, plus a giant flat-screen TV with a DVD player and a nice stereo. At one end was a fully stocked wet bar with tall stools by it—three of them—that abutted an enormous Jacuzzi. There was a big picture window at the other end through which we were treated to a lovely view of the mountains.

"That view will be really amazing at sunset," Tony exclaimed, enthralled.

We walked into the bedroom, and the first thing we noticed was the king-size bed in the center, covered in a soft down comforter and tons of pillows. One wall was mirrored, which I took in with a mischievous glint in my eye. There were beautiful stained-glass lamps on the bedside tables but otherwise no overhead lighting in the bedroom, which was fine with me. The dimmer the better, I figured.

Off the bedroom was a full spa bathroom with a huge bathtub, a giant stall shower, a beautifully tiled vanity, and even a bidet. We giggled at that. We were delighted to notice a small steam room beside the shower.

"Wow," I said to Tony as we walked back out into the sitting room.

"You said it," he replied, heading over to the bar. "Can I fix you a drink, my darling?"

"Please." I sank down into the plush sofa, thinking a drink was just what I needed to ease the tension in my shoulders and calm my slight nervousness.

Just as Tony brought me my Scotch and soda, there was a knock at the door. He smiled at me and went to answer it.

"Hi, Leslie!" Jenny exclaimed as she entered the sitting room. "Man, this room is excellent! I don't know if I've ever stayed anywhere as nice as this."

"I know. I don't think we have either. But fifteen years of marriage is no mean feat, so . . ."

Jenny nodded, and Tony asked her if she wanted a drink.

"Yeah, I think that's a great idea," she said. "Is there any red wine? Merlot or Cabernet? I'm not picky."

"Sure," Tony said, getting the corkscrew as Jenny took off her jacket and began unbuttoning her cardigan.

"I think I'll put on some music," I said, getting up and going over to fiddle with the electronic setup. Soon midtempo dance music filled the room. I walked back to the sofa, swaying my hips a little, and took a sip of my drink. Jenny was sipping her wine, and I saw that Tony had a glass of red as well. Seeing me moving to the music, Jenny stood up and started to sway a bit. Tony sat down on the floor with his glass to watch us dance.

"Should we put on a little show for you, babe?" I asked my husband, as though I didn't already know the answer. He nodded, and I moved closer to Jenny and put one hand on her hip. She ran a hand through her hair and then giggled a little, embarrassed. I brought my hand up from her hip to her cheek, and she looked me in the eye. I smiled. "We're just having fun here. No pressure," I assured her.

She nodded and took a sip of wine. I put my hand back on her hip and swayed a little closer to her, and she responded by putting an arm around my waist and moving her hips with mine. The song got a little faster, and we began moving in time to the music in rhythm with each other. Soon we were feverishly dancing, having put our drinks down on the coffee table, and we left our inhibitions behind.

When the song ended and a slow one began, Jenny and I moved close and began a sensual slow dance together. I glanced at Tony, who was still drinking his wine and gazing at us, transfixed. I also noticed that his jeans looked tighter in the front and made a mental note to relieve him of that discomfort once we finished dancing.

At that moment I looked back up. Jenny had lowered her head at that moment, so that we found ourselves eye to eye, and we held it for a moment. She must have sensed that I was ready, because she leaned down slightly and just touched her lips to mine. It was a simple, almost shy gesture, but it hit me like a bolt of lightning, sending waves of electric pleasure through my whole body. Her lips were so soft! She started to move away, but I held her there and kissed her for real, parting my lips a bit. The song almost entirely forgotten, Jenny took this opportunity to tentatively push the tip of her tongue into my mouth. This sent a second wave through me, and we began kissing in earnest, her lips and mine slowly moving over each other, tasting and tantalizing with every breath.

After a few moments of watching his wife and a beautiful redhead sensuously kissing, Tony must have grown tired of being a spectator, because suddenly there he was, behind me, softly rubbing his now-full erection against my ass. I moaned softly, feeling like I might burst from the pleasure of it. And we were still all fully dressed!

That reminded me that I'd meant to help Tony out with the tightness in his pants, so I reached behind me and unbuttoned and unzipped his jeans. Taking this as a cue that it was time for us all to be less encumbered by our clothing, Tony reached around and began unbuttoning my blouse even as I moved my hands to the bottom of Jenny's T-shirt and pulled it up and over her head. Standing there in her lacy pink bra, she reached behind me and lifted Tony's shirt over his head, and then he let my blouse fall down my arms, revealing the black bustier I'd bought specially for the occasion.

"Oh . . ." Tony breathed. "You're both so beautiful, I . . . I—"

"He doesn't know what to say. He's speechless!" I giggled, then turned and kissed him. He swatted my ass in a playful spank, and soon we were all laughing and horsing around with one another till we were in a heap on one of the sofas, with me in the middle.

After a moment things got serious again as Tony began kissing me. He moved his hand over my face, then down to my breasts, where his thumb found my nipple and began teasing it deliciously. Jenny took this opportunity to unzip my pants and reach her hand down inside, where her fingers were welcomed with warm wetness.

"Oh, Leslie," she murmured, pushing first one and then another finger into my moist center.

"Oh, Jenny," I moaned back, feeling the pleasure of two mouths and two sets of hands on my body. Tony had unclasped my bra and taken it off, and his lips and tongue were working over each of my nipples in turn, sucking and teasing and licking, even occasionally softy biting the hard nubs. As he delighted me with his mouth, I reached my hand into his boxer briefs and lightly caressed his rigid cock. With my other hand, I had found one of Jenny's hard nipples and was moving over it in a circle, eliciting oohs and ahhs from the adorable redhead. Her fingers were hard at work, too, as she swirled them around inside me and then moved up to tickle the hard button that ached for attention.

Jenny moaned as I flicked her nipple, and then her mouth found mine again and we kissed passionately, our tongues dueling and teasing. She was concentrating solely on my clitoris now, rubbing around it with just the right amount of pressure as Tony sucked at my nipples. I had taken firmer hold of his cock by now and was stroking it just the way I knew he liked it, rubbing in the drops of fluid that appeared on the tip.

"Oh, I'm close, I'm—" Tony's eyes locked on mine even as his tongue danced over my nipple, and Jenny's stroking became even more urgent. I tightened my grip on the base of Tony's cock, wanting to make sure he didn't come with me so I could savor his orgasm later. But I couldn't hold out anymore as the waves of electricity coursed through my body and my two lovers pleased me in perfect rhythm with each other. "I'm coming—oh, oh God, oh, I'm—" My whole body went rigid in climax, and as Tony watched, Jenny kissed me hard with her open mouth, her tongue plunging inside as her fingers plunged inside my vagina, the walls contracting in sweet release.

"Ohh, wow," I moaned softly as the last spasms shook through me. "That was . . ."

"She's speechless!" Tony laughed, clapping his hands. "That was beautiful, babe. You're beautiful."

"You are, Leslie. Your body is wonderful," Jenny smiled, pulling her hand from my panties and unselfconsciously licking her fingers. "Mmm. You taste good, too."

"I'd like to taste you, too, Jenny, but first I think I need to clean up a bit," I said, noticing how sticky I felt.

"Wait, though, babe," Tony said, his gaze shifting to the picture window. "Look at that!"

I turned my head just in time to see the sun disappearing behind the distant mountains, the sky awash in pink and gold. "That's just . . . gorgeous," I sighed.

We sat in silence for a few minutes, catching our breath and sipping our drinks, watching as the sunset lit the sky on fire and then slowly dimmed to a pinkish purple and the stars began to show through the night sky.

I got up then and went through the bedroom to the bathroom to pee and wash up. I looked at myself in the mirror and smiled.

My hair was a mess and my cheeks and chest were pink, but I did look awfully good. I look happy, I decided. And I was.

I wasn't surprised to find Tony and Jenny on the gigantic bed when I walked out of the bathroom. They, like me, had removed the rest of their clothing and were kissing tentatively, sitting on the edge of the bed.

"Hi," I said, joining them there.

"Hi," they said at the same time, each reaching out a hand and pulling me to them.

"I must taste you," Jenny said, pushing me back onto the bed and moving between my legs. "I can't wait any longer." With that, she began kissing my thighs and belly, running her fingers through my pubic hair. It felt wonderful.

Tony moved himself so that he was next to me and looked into my eyes. "You seem to be enjoying yourself," he said, smiling.

I kissed him softly. "I am, so much. Are you?"

"Oh, yeah," he said, reaching up and massaging my breast with his hand. I drew in my breath at that moment, not so much from Tony's hand on my breast but because Jenny had pushed her tongue inside me and it felt absolutely marvelous. I sighed, feeling like I must be the luckiest woman on earth.

Jenny moved her tongue in and out of me for a moment, then settled on my clit, circling it with her soft tongue again and again as my husband and I kissed passionately. "Honey," I said, "scoot up so that I can suck you."

Tony sure can move fast when he has motivation! His cock was in my mouth in a flash, the bulbous head pushing past my lips as I stretched my tongue to tickle his balls. "Oh, yeah, babe, that's perfect," Tony sighed, thrilled that his penis was finally getting some attention. I moved up and down his shaft with my tongue, loving the feeling of his hot erection as it tapped the back of my throat, then circling the head as I moved almost all the way back. Even as I was loving Tony orally, Jenny was hitting my sweet spot over and over, eating me with wild abandon. Her mouth was even more talented than her fingers, if that was possible.

After a few moments of this fabulous daisy chain, I thought I would go mad if I didn't get Tony's penis inside me. I was also aching to taste Jenny, who was wriggling her ass around as though she desperately needed some between-the-legs attention. So I stopped sucking Tony, gently moved away from Jenny's talented mouth, and suggested we switch it up a bit.

"I need you inside me," I told my husband, getting up onto all fours on the magnificent bed. "And you," I said, eyeing Jenny. "I've got to sample your juice, gorgeous. I bet it's divine."

"Oh, thank goodness," Jenny giggled. "I'm on fire!" She moved to lie beneath me with her upper body on the pillows and her lower half strategically beneath my face.

As Tony stood up, I told Jenny, "You smell great." Admiring her ginger bush, I added, "and you're a natural redhead! And all these freckles . . ." And with that, I began kissing all across her belly and thighs, savoring her beautiful skin. I moved my tongue down into her soft pubic hair and swirled it around, wanting to tease her a little bit. And it was working. Soon she was straining her legs and trying to push herself up into my mouth. Finally, I sank my tongue down into her wetness.

"Ohhh," I moaned, so thrilled with my first taste of her. She was so wet, so ready for my loving tongue.

"Oh, yes," Tony sighed. He was just standing, transfixed, as he watched his loving wife going down on the lovely Jenny. He had his cock in his hand and his other hand on my butt, and when he noticed me look up at him from between Jenny's legs, he moved his hand down between my ass cheeks to my wet inner lips and began stroking me.

"Oh, yeah," I moaned against Jenny's clit, which I was now lapping at lovingly. And then I felt Tony's cock at my entrance, and I stopped moving over Jenny for a moment as I savored the feeling of him as he sank into me to the hilt in one thrust. "Oh," I said, letting out a long breath.

It didn't take long for us to establish a good rhythm, me licking and sucking at Jenny and reveling in the noises she was making, encouraging me as the bucking of her hips became faster and more urgent, while Tony rammed in and out of me, slowly at first but gaining momentum as his balls slapped against me.

"Oh!" he shouted, smacking my ass, and I knew he was close to his climax, so I reached one hand down and began tugging on my clitoris as I flicked my tongue even faster over Jenny's. "Oh!" he exclaimed again, using his hips to piston his cock in and out of me desperately.

"Leslie, oh, Leslie, I'm close," Jenny breathed, running her hands through my hair as I plunged two fingers into her dripping opening. And then Jenny was coming, clamping her thighs on my face as she spasmed around my fingers. I held my mouth very still on her clit as she came, letting her ride it out. Before she was even done shaking, Tony cried, "Oh! Les, oh!" and smacked my ass once more as he made one final plunge into me, staying inside and spurting deep, murmuring happily as his pleasure ran out of him and into me. Feeling him surging into me, and swirling my fingers around my clit, I came last, falling onto Jenny's belly as wave after wave of glorious feeling came over me.

Tony withdrew and lay down beside Jenny and me on the bed. We were all panting and glistening with sweat, utterly spent and smiling blissfully. I looked up at Jenny and kissed her breast, then rolled over to embrace my husband.

"I love you," Tony murmured into my ear.

"Happy anniversary, my love," I whispered.

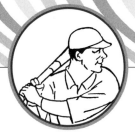

The Boys of Summer

Toni de la Salle

The smell of fresh-cut grass, the sound of bat hitting ball, the taste of a hot dog—all these things mean summer to me. Oh, and the sight of those fit men in their tight baseball uniforms.

I've always been a sucker for a baseball player. I don't understand why. Maybe it's all those things, maybe it's the gloves they wear with those long fingers, maybe it's the cups that make their organs seem so much more prodigious than those of mere mortal men. Something about them gets me wet.

So it was not unusual to find me there, after an amateur game on a Tuesday night, down at the local park. The out-of-towners had beaten my hometown boys by a solid margin, and two of the muscular boys from Deaneville had caught my eye. I figured I could get one of them.

Was I in for a shock.

They had gathered their gear and were headed for their cars when I stepped into the entry of the dugout. I caught both of their hot gazes traveling the shape of my body, and I smiled wickedly at them. "Hi, I'm Marnie," I purred.

They both smiled back, and the white one was the first to recover his tongue. "I'm Brett. This is Stan." His gesture took in the black man on his right. I let my eyes take in both of them and let them see me looking.

Brett had surfer-boy good looks. He was tall and skinny with an underlying musculature that just made you want to lick every drop of sweat from his body. Stan was shorter and more compact with something of a dangerous look to him. He looked thicker throughout, and I had trouble taking my eyes off of his well-muscled thighs. They both had big hands. My wicked smile became a little wider.

I waved my hand before my face. "A little hot out here, don't you think?"

Stan's deep voice came out. "It just got a little hotter."

"Well," I gasped, "let's do something about that."

They followed eagerly as I led the way into a nearby equipment shack. I closed the door behind us and switched on the light before turning the deadbolt that would protect us from intrusion. My feet skipped over to them, and my hands worked on their crotches.

I grinned as I found both men of proper thickness and hardness. My fingers worked at their belts as they tugged off their shirts. When their belts were undone and their pants unsnapped and unzipped, I dug my hands into their jockstraps, my hands filling with throbbing man. I leaned forward and kissed Stan's thick lips, then Brett's. They both moaned appropriately as I stroked them. I felt Brett's hand working at the button on my shorts. He undid it and unzipped them before sliding his hand in.

He grunted as his fingers encountered my shorn pubis, not the expected feel of panties. Undaunted, he slid his hand farther in and down to cup my silky slit. His middle finger parted my labia and found my clit, then my opening. He massaged them both deftly while my tongue pushed its way into his mouth.

Stan, meanwhile, had moved in behind me. His hands had pushed my shirt up and unhooked the skimpy lace bra I wore. His fingertips found my erect nipples and began to do wonderful things to them. His lips caressed the nape of my neck while his teeth nibbled there.

We all stopped at the same time to finish removing our clothes. We three stood there in glorious nudity, breathless anticipation dawning in all of us, before we attacked one another.

Brett's kisses were insistent as his long, slender prick pressed into my stomach. Stan's shorter but thicker dick pressed between my ass cheeks as his hands gripped and massaged my tits. I turned to face my other lover.

His strong arms wrapped around me, and he lifted me from the ground. I wrapped my legs around his waist and snaked my hand between us to direct his erection into my wet and wanting opening. The head of his magnificent cock plugged hard into my hole, and I grunted in exquisite sensation. As I sank onto him, he began to rut madly, pushing it farther into me. It stretched me open as I took all seven inches into my waiting void. I felt full of man and worried a little that I wouldn't be able to feel Brett's in my sweet vagina when Stan was done.

I didn't know that such a worry was misplaced. Brett had no intention of filling my vagina. His big, strong hands gripped my ass cheeks as he pushed them apart. He crouched behind me and pressed the head of his slender dong against my anus. I could feel that hole opening as he increased the pressure. That familiar pop in my head signaled that he was inside, and he slowly continued his advance into me. He didn't stop until I could feel his balls directly under me, and I knew that all nine of his slender inches were stuffed in my rectum. I had the random thought that both Brett's and Stan's scrotums were pressed against each other as they were both sunk in my body to the hilt. They didn't seem to care.

We rested there for a few seconds, both of my studs buried in my body. It was a delicious sensation that I didn't think could be equaled.

Then they started to do me.

Stars exploded in my head as they held me still and thrust merrily away in my holes. I could hear the scream from my throat as they ravished me. Their cocks were like red-hot pokers firing into my body but spreading sweet pleasure rather than pain. The sweat dripped into my eyes and onto their hips as they continued to pound away. A small part of my intellect noted that this couldn't be the first time they'd shared a woman like this. I wondered for a second how many women had been clutched in this embrace, how lucky I was to be one of them.

Then all thought stopped as my first orgasm tore through me. It was actually unexpected, but it was thoroughly real, as was the animal scream of absolute joy that was ripped from my lips. I squeezed them with my holes, but they didn't slow for a moment, their thrusts making me more sensitive to the intense pleasure of this sex. I all but collapsed in their arms, but they continued to hold me still, continued to go at me still.

My consciousness ebbed for a moment, but a second orgasm, stronger than the first, fried my nerves. They continued to wash over me. Never had I been so full, never had I felt so good. Never had I felt so much a woman as I did while Stan and Brett drove their powerful rods into me.

Suddenly, Brett froze and then drove himself in with one final, savage thrust. I could feel the hot semen from him spurt into me. It burned powerfully as it flowed into my bowels. Stan similarly drove in again, and I could feel his seed filling my womb. And with that sensation, the dam broke.

I wailed with pleasure, laughing and crying as a final orgasm washed over me. This time, consciousness completely left me.

I awoke on my side. A blanket was under me and my head was on Brett's leg. Stan held me from behind. I didn't know how long we had been there or if they were asleep. It didn't take long to find out the latter, though.

I shifted and could feel Stan's hot meat move against my ass. It was sore from the earlier dicking, but Stan hardened there anyway. Part of me really liked that thought. I glanced up and saw Brett's shriveled member. I licked my lips as he shifted, recognizing the light in my eyes. My hand came up and I gripped him, already hardening for another round, too.

As I slurped his dick into my mouth, I could feel Stan starting to work his thick prick into my anus. He had the head there but was having trouble pushing it in. I pushed back against him and saw stars again when the head pushed in. I focused on sucking Brett's cock, which had reached full size. I wrapped a hand around the base and licked his throbbing head like a lollipop. He groaned his pleasure as I took the head into my mouth and sucked, the heady mixture of the taste of ass and semen seeping into my mouth. I gently grated my teeth against the underside, and his eyes widened.

Meanwhile, Stan's balls now rested against my dripping snatch. My ass, which was no stranger to dicks, had never been opened so wide. I bucked myself against him, impatient for it, and he began to stroke his dick in and out of me. I ran my lips up and down on Brett's slick cock with the same rhythm.

As Stan increased the force of his strokes, I also increased the depth of mine on Brett. Finally, Stan wasn't holding back. And each time his balls smacked my snatch, Brett's dong slid into my throat. I felt them both seize at the same time and smiled inside.

Stan's balls emptied into my intestines just as Brett's drained into my esophagus. I could again feel that exquisite fire burn in my body as my two lovers climaxed inside of me. And from their grunts and moans of pleasure, I knew that I'd given them both the same joy they'd given me.

They dressed, and I shooed them out so that I could arrange my own clothes again. I promised to call them next time I was in Deaneville, and they promised the same treatment when they returned here. Neither hesitated to kiss me deeply before they departed, and I know it was with real affection that both fondled my naked breasts before they left.

So I dressed alone. I balled up the blanket and threw it into a corner, where I'll be able to use it next time I bring someone to the equipment shed. Hmmm, come to think of it, our boys have a game next week . . . against those Deaneville Demons. I think it's time for a road trip.

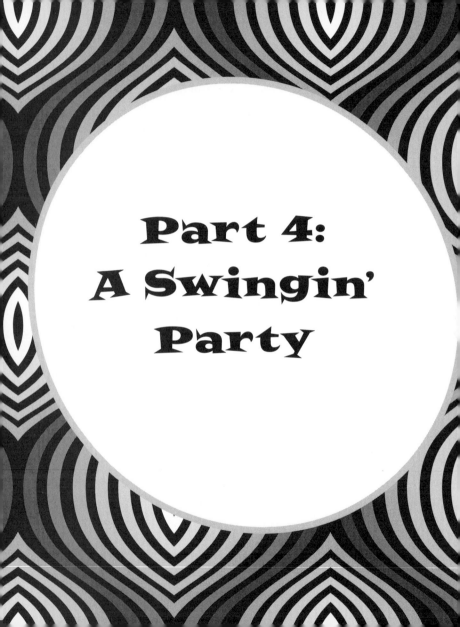

Part 4:
A Swingin’
Party

*Sex between two people is a beautiful thing;
between five, it's fantastic.*

—*Woody Allen*

Y ou might think it's safe to assume that all the information you need for group sex can be found in Part 3 on threesomes, and it's true that a lot of the rules and caveats overlap. But there are lots of things we haven't covered yet in the world of multiple sexual partners, and lots of things from the previous section won't apply to swinging.

LISTEN UP, THIS IS IMPORTANT

Moving from one-on-one sex or even threesomes to group sex is like leaving your Cape Cod house in the suburbs for Vegas.

In general, the vibe surrounding swinging and swapping is very different from that associated with threesomes. For one thing, swinging usually occurs among two or more couples, which means that there's less of a chance that someone will end up being the odd man (or woman) out.

Plus there are couples who would never consider adding more than one other person to their sex life and couples that think just one extra person wouldn't be fair.

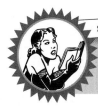

SECRETS TO MAKE YOU LOOK GOOD

See, adding extra people to the bed just means you're being thoughtful.

The differences between threesomes and larger groups will be investigated a little later in this part, but for now, let's just celebrate the fact that there are so many options.

SNAP OF THE FINGER

Feeling left out in threesomes? Simply even out the number of participants.

This section touches on some of the preliminary stages of acquainting yourself with the lifestyle but generally takes the tack that if you're getting into swinging and swapping, you may already be pretty well acquainted. If that's not the case or if there are more questions than we've provided answers for here, go back and look at Part 3 again.

First some basics and then a quick history of swinging and swapping before we move on to the juicer stuff.

A SWINGIN' GLOSSARY

There are a few terms to add to the glossary in Part 3, too. The following will help further your understanding of the swinging lifestyle:

* **BUKKAKE:** A sexual practice in which several men take turns ejaculating on one person, usually a woman who is kneeling in the center of the circle.
* **EXHIBITIONISM:** Engaging in sexual activity alone or with someone other than your partner while your partner and/or others watch.
* **FULL SWAP:** Engaging in penetrative intercourse with a person or people besides your partner in a swinging situation.

* **GANGBANG:** A sexual situation in which one person has sex with many other people; the main person may be a man or a woman, and the people he or she has sex with generally do not engage in sexual contact with one another.
* **GROUP SEX:** A general term for multiple sexual encounters occurring in the same location.
* **HOT WIFE:** Describes a practice in which a woman has sex with a partner or partners who are not her husband while her husband and perhaps others watch.

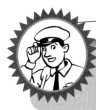

YOU'RE WELCOME FOR THE TIP

It's fine and dandy to brag about your spouse by calling her your hot wife; however, just make sure you're not in a swinger's bar first.

* **POLYAMORY:** A term used to describe a situation in which more than two people are involved in a love relationship; polyamorous folks generally object to being called swingers.
* **SOFT SWAP:** Sexual activity with multiple partners involving kissing, touching, and oral sex.

SWINGING: A BRIEF HISTORY

Lots of folks in "the lifestyle" credit the ancient Romans and Greeks as the inspiration for their multipartnered sexual proclivities, but the actual practice of swinging as we know it today began in the twentieth century.

The ancient Greeks held *órgia* (where the word "orgy" comes from), which were religious ceremonies that only initiates could attend. The fact that these rites were held at night and were secretive led to speculation that all sorts of naughtiness were afoot.

Folks who've done extensive research on the subject believe that swinging began in the 1950s in military communities. This relatively small community practice, called simply wife swapping at the time, gave way to the explosion of the sexual revolution in the 1960s, and then all bets were off.

Suddenly, organizations dedicated to the practice of swinging started popping up. The first was the Sexual Freedom League, which was founded in 1963 in New York City with the advertised purpose of promoting sexuality among its members and advocating for change in the way the government dealt with sexual issues. They often had "nude parties," but that was really just a euphemism for orgies.

From there it was a short step to the North American Swing Club Association, now known as NASCA International, a California organization dedicated to providing accurate information about the lifestyle and clubs and events you can go to. They even publish a guide you can buy at your local bookstore (but the store may have to order it) or purchase online.

Depending on what study you look at, anywhere between 5 and 50 percent of married couples engage in swinging of some sort. Indeed, reported figures of the lifestyle community are that anywhere between 3 million and 4 million people practice swinging worldwide.

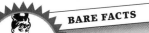

Swingers' ages average in the forties, and a majority who choose to talk about the practice generally report that it improves their relationships either by making the participants more open about sex with one another or by curbing cheating behavior. Swingers are generally middle class, white, and married.

There is a new practice afoot among swingers, called selective swinging, which tends to feature younger, more attractive people in more upscale venues. Instead of 1980s hair and 1970s morality, which is what most of us picture when we think of swinging—admit it—think elegant, sophisticated, social sexuality with gourmet food and expensive liquor. As happens with all things, marketing folks have gotten involved, which means that even swinging is fashionable somewhere. If it's your thing, celebrate!

THREESOMES VERSUS LARGER GROUPS

Although threesomes fall under the umbrella of group sex, they are very different from the practice generally known as swinging, in which mainly couples participate. Swinging has more of a playful, party feel to it than threesome play does, and not only because there are more participants. Threesomes seem to be taken more seriously in a relationship, whereas swing parties are just that: the play is celebratory, and there isn't too much worry—at least on the surface—about the consequences group sex will have on couples' relationships. There is a strong community atmosphere with swinging and larger groups; indeed, folks who participate in large couples' parties are there for the sex, but they're also there for the companionship and the laughs.

Unlike with threesomes, in which it is helpful to be bisexual or at least bicurious, with swinging in larger groups you needn't have any bisexual encounters at all. That's not to say it doesn't happen; it's just rarer. And if it does happen, it's generally between or among women.

There is certainly a fundamental numerical divide between swinger play and threesome play, too: the numbers just don't work out the same. Whereas with swing clubs and parties it is generally all couples, threesome events don't work if there aren't singles as well. Singles are sometimes accepted at swingers' parties, and whether they are or not should usually be specified explicitly in whatever literature you have about the event.

Don't worry, though: whichever you participate in, there's no shortage of places to go to meet interested partners or couples. NASCA reports events in forty-three of the fifty United States, and some of those venues are even threesome-centric.

Make no mistake, though; swing events are the more publicized of the two, and you can basically pick any niche you want and find other folks who'll go to a party for it with you. From enormous events such as "SwingFest: the world's largest swingers party and convention" to more outdoorsy parties such as SwingStock (a four-day campout event that attracts hundreds of people to Minnesota every summer), there's bound to be something that fits your group sex needs.

YOU'RE WELCOME FOR THE TIP

SwingStock parties include no swimsuit competitions, but do offer theme dances, games, barbecues, and a chance to catch up with old friends and have sex with them.

But before you screw up your courage, so to speak, and register for an event, you might want to ask yourself a few questions.

SHOULD YOU SWING?

If you're considering a trip to Swingertown, safety needs to be your primary concern. We're talking here about physical safety as well as the emotional kind, which we'll get to in a minute. Ensuring your physical safety means you must always use condoms to prevent AIDS and other STDs as well as unwanted pregnancies. For this second consideration, a backup method should also be used unless all the female participants are past menopause. (This kind of party happens more often than you might think.)

Also make sure you go to a club or party that is vouched for in some way either by NASCA or another organization or by a friend or acquaintance to make sure the folks you're meeting aren't into drugs or violent behavior. They are strangers, after all, and you're at your most vulnerable when you are naked, never mind how open you are when you're about to have an orgasm! Just play it safe.

LISTEN UP, THIS IS IMPORTANT

Take care of yourself at swinger functions and clubs the way you would at any event, only more so, since you probably won't be wearing any underwear . . . or clothing, for that matter.

Those are the practical, tangible things you need to be sure about before you take the plunge into group sex, and they're pretty easy to tackle. What might not be so easy are the intangible considerations that must go into your decision whether to go this route. Within your relationship, you must be able to discuss sex openly and honestly. If you're unable to talk frankly about what goes on between you when you're nude together, don't even think about swinging. If the level of openness required is completely beyond you, you should try reading erotica aloud together or watching porn or talking about fantasies or reading Part 2 of this book to each other or any number of things to get you comfortable with your sex life before even considering adding other people to it.

COMMUNICATION

Assuming you and your partner are comfortable chatting it up on all things sexual, move on to asking yourselves some questions.

Quiz for Couples Who Are Contemplating Swinging

- ❏ We are committed to each other and secure in our relationship.

- ❏ We are open about our sexual fantasies and share them with each other.

- ❏ One or both of us fantasizes about having sex with multiple partners.

- ❏ Neither of us is a jealous person.

- ❏ We can separate our loving relationship from sex.

- ❏ Experimenting sexually is very important to both of us.

- ❏ Each of us would enjoy seeing our partner being pleased by someone else.

- ❏ If we try something new sexually and it's not great for one or both of us, we can get past it.

- ❏ We are both able to have sex without getting emotionally involved.

- ❏ We have no trouble communicating with each other about what we want in the bedroom.

The more of these statements you checked off, the more ready you are to get involved with the lifestyle, but no quiz in a book can really tell you if you're ready to open your relationship to this type of sexual encounter. What you must do is really talk to each other, do some research, and make sure it's something you both want to do. Keep in mind these considerations as you discuss it:

* Both members of the couple must be into swinging or having group sex. Neither should have to talk the other into the experience.

* Though some studies report that a majority of swingers say the group thing is beneficial to their marriages or even that swinging has saved their marriages, there is no definitive proof of this. It may help, but it may not.

* There's no going back after you do it. Once you and your partner have had sex with other people at a swing party or another couple's home, it's done, and your relationship will be different.

Other Considerations

Of course your first thoughts when considering a foray into group sex should be how it will affect your relationship with your partner and how you will stay physically safe, but there are other considerations as well.

Practicality is one of them. There's a reason swinging is often referred to as "the lifestyle." It is, in fact, *a way of living* for many of those who participate in it, which means it takes up a lot of time and energy. Because of this, you may need to be able to tell people about it, such as family members or coworkers, and even in these progressive times, there will be those who will not be understanding and/or supportive. If you have children, as many swingers do, you may need to consider what you will tell them or what you will do with them when you go to events or clubs or when you want to have a grown-up play date in your home.

A woman's role in group sex and its social implications is another consideration for those about to swing. Many argue that women are objectified in an objectionable way in group sexual practices, especially activities such as bukkake and gangbanging, in which one woman is often the central sexual outlet for several different men.

Others say swinging empowers women sexually by allowing couples to engage in sexual fact-finding together in a way that makes sex not so gender-specific; that is, they are able to engage in sexual practices they find appealing or satisfying solely on the basis of arousal and not on any standards set by society (for example, others' morality or spousal duty). Those who are in favor of swinging say it levels the playing field for men and women, so to speak.

Either way, some women might like to surrender control or might find it liberating in its own way to be the centerpiece of a sexual encounter for so many men, and some might not. Some women who swing might not engage in gangbanging or bukkake, preferring instead a regular swap or filling the role of a hot wife in that scenario. Regardless, it must be up to the woman herself to decide, and she needn't do anything she doesn't want to do.

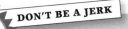

DON'T BE A JERK

A central tenet of swinging for men and women is to do what you want as long as no one gets hurt who doesn't want to. "No" means "no" *all* the time.

YES!

After you've discussed all the pros and cons and decided you and your partner would like to try group sex, you'll have to figure out what kind of situation you want and what kind of couple or group you'll be most comfortable with or attracted to or any other criteria you may have. You'll also need to decide how many other people you want to swing with, and that's a very personal decision. It seems prudent to start small and then work your way up, but really, it's up to you and your partner.

But once that's done, there are several ways you can go about meeting other couples with whom to get naked. You'll just need to find willing folks. Here's where to look:

✳ *Your friends and neighbors.* Lots of folks get started in swinging fairly innocently with friends they get together with socially. Drinks lead to flirting, which leads to naked fun together. Do it if you're comfortable with it, but your relationship will change, no doubt about it.

SECRET TIP

Swinging with friends and neighbors can get dicey if only because you might never again want to look them in the eye after you've looked them in the crotch.

✳ *Lifestyle clubs.* These are swingers' clubs in which couples can go to check one another out and then all play together. Not all clubs allow sex, though, so make sure you know which kind you are in: on-premises (for the sex) or off-premises (for just the meeting). The major bonus with these clubs is that your first introduction is face to face; you won't have to worry that they won't show up. The drawback is that there isn't a lifestyle club in every city or town, so you might have to travel a bit to find one. Luckily, NASCA International can keep you apprised of events in your area. Which brings us to . . .

✳ *NASCA's published guide.* This provides comprehensive listings of clubs, parties, conventions, publications, and holidays for "those who want more than just one bite." It's really your first stop on the road to finding your ideal swinging situation.

* *Swing publications.* This is where you'll find personal ads detailing any situation you could wish for. This is a good resource for a couple that wants to swing with just one other couple in a private setting because, for example, they are not comfortable in a club with all that nudity. Often the publication will have photos and other useful information to help you decide on the Smiths or the Joneses.

* *The Internet.* There are so many adult dating sites online it would take years to list them, but those such as *adultfriendfinder.com* and *adultfindout.com* are popular and allow you to specify exactly what you want. They're also generally free. If you want to keep it very local and you're in a fairly large metropolitan area, a good place to try is your city's alternative newsweekly's personals page. These pages have tons of ads for folks seeking all manner of kinky fun. The drawbacks with adult personal ads are the same as those with regular ones: People lie. The couple you choose might not be "extremely attractive" or even passable, or they might not show up. It might also take some time to find a couple because there are apparently millions of swingers out there looking to play. But you've already committed to spending quite a bit of time on this, so don't let that deter you.

BOUNDARIES

Although the swinging community is a pretty open one, boundaries must be set and respected, just as in threesomes. There is perhaps less of this in larger groups, mainly because a couple is not sharing one other person, so jealousy may be less of an issue.

Swinging couples *do* have jealousy issues, of course; however, it's just that he or she may be too busy also having sex with another person at the very same time, and so he or she will be pleasantly distracted.

Before you and your partner attend a club, event, or party or before you meet a couple you've selected in another way, discuss what you want to happen, what each of you is allowed to do, anything you might not be comfortable seeing your partner doing, and any other concerns you may have about the specific acts that will be performed. You might feel that this takes the fun or playfulness out of the experience, but it's important to remember what Germaine Greer said: "No sex is better than bad sex." Not respecting other people's boundaries, including those of your partner, can make for some pretty bad sex. So set boundaries before your first swinging experience—and adjust them on subsequent experiences—and follow those rules.

ESSENTIAL SWINGING ETIQUETTE

Some helpful hints to make your first—and subsequent, should you so choose—group sex party a smashing success:

✳ If you're going to a club, make sure you know whether it's on- or off-premises. That's really important. If you're not supposed to get naked and have sex in the club, you shouldn't do it, and you'll feel like a real jerk if you do. Likewise, if you think you're just going to a place to get a feel for what happens and end up getting an actual feel, you might also feel like a jerk.

* If you're going to someone's home for a party, ask in advance what kinds of activities will occur or if there is a theme of some sort and if you can bring anything—just like at a regular dinner party or potluck.

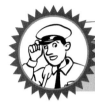

YOU'RE WELCOME FOR THE TIP

If attending a swinging potluck, your dish will be the only thing in the room that's covered.

* Arrive showered and well groomed. For obvious reasons, fingernails and pubic hair should be trimmed.
* Arrive with your partner at a couples-only party. You might also decide that the two of you will stay together the whole time at your first party. It's not a bad idea, especially the first time. It's up to you to decide how you will handle future parties if you choose to keep going with the lifestyle.
* Apprise yourself of the alcohol policy at a particular event, whether it's at a club or a private party, and abide by that policy.
* Bring your own personal items, such as towels or lubricants, or ask if they will be provided. A robe might not be a bad idea, either.
* As with any sexual situation, toys and accessories can be a welcome addition. These may include vibrators, lubricants (highly recommended), blindfolds, or any other accoutrements you might enjoy. Just make sure everyone's on board.
* It cannot be stressed enough: Condoms and dental dams are a must!
* Keep liquor to a minimum. Avoid drugs entirely.
* You're allowed to turn people down, but try to be sensitive about it. They're swinging people, sure, but they still have feelings.

✳ If something happens that you don't enjoy or that makes you feel uncomfortable, let it be known without unnecessarily hurting someone's feelings or spoiling the mood. In other words, try to be frank and polite at the same time. Everyone's needs at and expectations of a party are different, so it is best not to assume anything about the other guests.

SNAP OF THE FINGER

Remember these items whether you're going to a party or hosting your own:

- ✳ Lube
- ✳ Open mind
- ✳ Sense of humor
- ✳ Respect
- ✳ More lube
- ✳ Healthy body image
- ✳ Adventurous spirit
- ✳ Condoms
- ✳ Energy
- ✳ Lube

LUBE REVISITED

You'll need a lot of lubrication for an evening or weekend of group sex. No matter how much natural lubrication a woman may produce, even if she's above average, you will need more. This is an unequivocal fact. See page 12 for the whole scoop on lubrication.

AFTER THE FIRST TIME

Sometime after your first swing or group sex party (though probably not immediately afterward because you're likely to fall asleep thirty seconds after your last orgasm), you and your partner must talk about the encounter.

Here are some questions to ask yourself and each other:

* Did both of us get what we wanted out of it?
* Did we enjoy ourselves?
* Did any part of it make us feel uncomfortable or bad?
* What feelings besides arousal did we experience?
* If we were to do it again, are there things we would do differently?
* Do we want to do it again?
* What did we learn about own sexuality?
* What did each of us learn about his or her partner's sexuality?

The answers to these questions will help you decide if you want to make group sex a regular part of your sexual repertoire or if once was enough to satisfy your urge and curiosity. Your feelings about the experience may change, so keep talking about it as that happens. If nothing else comes of your swinging experience, you will have learned to talk openly about sex with your partner, and that is an extremely important skill.

Assuming you've met some folks you like playing with and you've decided after your first encounter that you'd like to swing some more—and you enjoy entertaining, of course—you might want to host your own parties.

TIPS FOR HOSTING YOUR OWN PARTY

* Don't spend so much time hosting that you forget that you're there to have a good time, too. At a certain point, relinquish your duties, strip off that G-string, and join the fun!
* Designate certain rooms for certain activities. For example, your living room can be the social room, where guests eat and drink and talk but don't necessarily have sex. Your den could serve as the

open-play room, where folks can feel free to get it on with other folks watching. You might designate your guest room as a private room for those with less exhibitionistic tendencies. Make sure to let your guests know if any rooms are off limits, such as your bedroom or your kids' bedrooms.

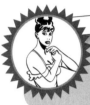

BARE FACTS

Speaking of your kids, it might be best if they weren't home for this. Make arrangements for them to spend the night elsewhere, preferably in the next county.

✳ Clean up. This should go without saying, right? It's like any other party, right? You want to make a good impression. But since guests will often be naked and doing *very* personal things with one another, cleanliness is even more of an issue.

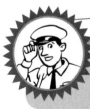

YOU'RE WELCOME FOR THE TIP

Use antibacterial disinfectant for the cleanup and have fresh sheets on hand for when it's time to actually sleep.

✳ Make sure your guests know what your policy is on hot-button issues such as alcohol, drugs, and condoms.
✳ Have a theme party. Sure, swinging is a fine theme in itself, but it might be fun to come up with a creative concept to distinguish yourself as a premier party host and hostess.

FIVE FUN PARTIES TO HOST

Speaking of theme parties, here are five of the easiest and most fun to host.

Costume Party

This isn't too tough: just inform your guests that the party is "fancy-dress," which can mean evening gowns and tuxes or dressing up in costume, whichever you prefer. You can have a masquerade ball, with masks, too.

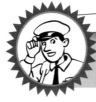

As far as costumes go, you can let it be a free-for-all or designate a genre if you want. How about a 1980s party? Or 1960s? If all your guests are interested in similar things, it shouldn't be too difficult to find one for your theme. Renaissance or gothic clothing makes for interesting, sexy costumes. If everyone loves *Lord of the Rings*, try that (though cross your fingers that folks favor elves over trolls). Or have a famous faces of the 1950s party at which guests can be old-time movie stars such as

James Dean and Marilyn Monroe. You might decide that the costumes should be limited to people's undies so that no one knows who anyone is dressed as until later in the evening, after the regular clothes come off. The possibilities are endless. Just think of your guests and their interests and brainstorm. As with the sex, the only limit is your imagination.

Around-the-World Party

This is a swinging take on a favorite college dormitory game. Make each room in your home a different country, with nationality-specific refreshments and atmosphere in each—plus a sexy twist.

In France, guests sip French martinis and French kiss. Maybe there are even escargots. (Or maybe not, if slimy gastropods are not sexy to you.) Add some French pop music for a real—and amusing—treat.

In Russia, guests lounge on a luxurious faux-fur (or real, if you like) rug while drinking White Russians. They'll be lining up to use this room privately later on—there's nothing like naked skin against fur.

Travel to Mexico: take off that warm muffler (and some other clothing, if you want), don a serape, and enjoy a refreshing glass of sangria.

You get the idea. Pick your favorite countries and set them up in your own home. You needn't spend much money or time on props; a sketch of the Eiffel Tower is sufficient for France, maybe some orangey lighting and mariachi music for Mexico. The real fun is in the sexy details. But remember, you don't want any of your swingers to get too toasted, so keep the drinks weak.

SECRET TIP

If you don't want your swingers getting tipsy or drunk, be ironic and serve only virgin cocktails.

Old-School Key Party

You may remember that in the 1997 Ang Lee movie *The Ice Storm*, there was a key party after which Joan Allen has some very uncomfortable-looking sex in a tiny car to get back at her husband, Kevin Kline, who has been having an affair with Sigourney Weaver. Your key party needn't be anything like that, though if you can swing the swinging 1970s decor and outfits, go for it. (And if you can get movie stars to attend, more power to you!)

A key party basically works like this: each man puts his keys in a jar, and each woman chooses a set and goes home with that man. Or you might put each man's watch in the jar the way they did in that episode of *The O.C.* Or how about cell phones? The difference with your key party will be that no one will go home with anyone—the sex can happen right there! And ideally no one will have uncomfortable sex in a car (unless that's what they're into).

A party that is a throwback to the generation that started it all in terms of swinging—a homage to back in the day, if you will—doesn't need to seem dated or stale even if you decide the guests should dress in their best bell bottoms and platform shoes. It's entirely up to you. You can take the basic idea that everyone randomly selects and keeps a partner for the evening and do whatever you want with it. But for groups that have swung together before—and in which all the members are attracted to one another—this can add a spicy wild card to the party.

Potluck Party

Because swinging is a sexual activity *and* a social one, you might decide a swinging party is also a good time to enjoy wonderful homemade food. There's no reason for the only main course to be sex, right? You'll need your sustenance if you're going to keep going for hours anyway, and hors d'oeuvres alone won't cut it.

As far as the food goes, you can pick a theme for that if you want, too. You can do all vegetarian if your group goes that way, or tapas, or Asian fusion. Choose anything you like but make sure all the guests communicate what they're bringing so you don't have ten appetizers and no desserts or five different shrimp dishes. Dig in and enjoy—you'll need all the energy you can get!

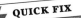

QUICK FIX

If you are serving food, set up some ground rules about whether it can be used for sex play. Either that or reserve a steam cleaner for the following day.

Aromatherapy Massage Party

For a laid-back evening, why not try an aromatherapy massage party? It's easy. Ask each couple or person to bring a different essential oil. Popular ones include grapefruit (for cleansing and purifying), lavender (for calming and balancing), peppermint (for stimulating), and jasmine (an aphrodisiac).

Each couple can take turns giving each other a massage using the oil—choices of massage include full-body, feet, hands, back, and head, but try to avoid genitals, at least at first. As everyone watches and you and your partner rub each other, everyone's sexual tension will build as they all become relaxed in their muscles and minds, which will make the sexual encounters to come truly explosive.

PARTY GAMES AND ICEBREAKERS

A theme for your party should diffuse any nervousness or tension on the part of your guests. However, if you think themes are too much work, too kitschy, or not your style but you'd like to liven things up a bit, try any of these exciting, enticing games and icebreakers:

* Dance. It eases tension and gets you loosened up. It can also make you feel sexy as you move your hips and sway to music.
* Play truth or dare. Start with truth questions and move on to more suggestive dares. Or play spin the bottle, starting with kissing and then moving on to more grown-up activities for a twist on everyone's favorite teenage party game.
* If you're in a group of seasoned swingers but they haven't all swung together before, go around the room for story time. Have each tag team tell the story of their first time swinging. That should get everyone laughing and comfortable sharing with one another.
* Play strip poker or strip something else. Strip Trivial Pursuit is a good one, since it is usually played with teams, so you and your partner will get undressed at the same pace—all the while showing off your knowledge of sports and leisure.

* Try some karaoke. Sure, it's embarrassing, but if folks are uncomfortable taking their clothes off right off the bat, perhaps some humiliation of the nonnaked variety will make the transition a little more palatable.
* Watch a sexy movie. When all else fails, try some porn.

QUICK FIX

If your guests are having trouble getting in the swinging mood, ask the exhibitionists in the group to put on a show for the rest of the guests. They will probably jump at the chance, and before you know it, a few hours later they all will be looking under couch cushions for their underwear.

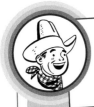

WELL, LOOK WHO FINALLY MADE THE
Rodeo

A lot of the information about threesomes is the same as that for group sex, but there are some **DIFFERENCES**. One of these is the vibe: swinging has more of a sense of **COMMUNITY**, whereas threesomes seem to be a more **PRIVATE** endeavor. Group sex is often referred to as "the lifestyle" for a reason: it takes up a lot of time in your life, and not everyone will be pleased to learn of your choice. In other words, it's not easy explaining your love of group sex at the family holiday reunion.

Stories

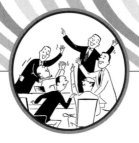

BOARDROOM

J. M. Thompson

Jerry had always been tempted to print up a new sign for the company boardroom, changing the name to Bored Room. Considering the way the meeting had started out, it looked like he was going to spend most of the morning trying to stay awake. It was well understood that the one unforgivable sin in the boardroom was to snore louder than the CEO during the meetings.

Rutherford B. Bodine had been well into his eighties when Jerry attended his first executive staff meeting more than five years earlier. Back then, Rutherford was actively in charge of the business, not the figurehead he had become in the last few years. The firm's president, Harold Bodine, Rutherford's nephew, actually ran the company and pretty much chaired the executive staff meetings. Although well known for his skinny-dipping into the secretarial pool, he did manage the company as well as or better than his uncle.

In preparation for the meeting, Jerry had guzzled several caffeinated soft drinks, so he didn't begin to fade until the meeting rolled into its third hour. By then Rutherford had been sleeping for about two hours and his snoring had generated a few waves of chuckles through the room. When Jerry dropped his pen onto his pad, he recognized he was not far from dropping off too, so he squirmed a bit in his chair and sat upright at the table. This worked for about five minutes before his eyes were slowly closing. . . .

He was abruptly awakened when Jen, the tall, auburn-haired head of marketing, stood up and shouted at Benjamin from procurement, "Ben, you haven't got the balls to support our effort."

Benjamin, a nervous, prematurely gray-haired man in his midthirties who had been sitting next to her, jumped up, turned to face her, and replied, "Of course I have the balls. You just—" He suddenly stopped speaking. Everyone in the room, including old Rutherford, who had also been awakened by the commotion, simply stared as Jen slowly squeezed her hand, which had a firm hold on Benjamin's crotch.

As he began to wince in pain, she said softly, "I guess I was wrong. You do have balls, Ben."

Without another word, without turning his head from her face, he reached up and in an attempt to gain a stronger negotiating position cupped his hand over her breast. While everyone watched, he gently squeezed first her left breast and then her right. Jen slowly moved her hand from his crotch and brushed his hands from her breasts. All the attendees prepared themselves for her to slap him; instead, she reached up, grabbed his head, and pulled it to her as she tilted her head and kissed him directly on the lips.

Harold Bodine immediately jumped to his feet, expecting them to stop, but the couple continued kissing, completely ignoring him. After watching them for a few minutes, he glanced over to his petite assistant, a young, statuesque woman with jet black hair, squinted a bit while thinking, and then turned to one of the junior associates sitting near the door and said, "Lock the door." He sat back down in his chair and rolled it over next to June, his assistant and obvious next conquest. Placing a hand on her knee, he began to negotiate some mutually beneficial benefits as Jerry looked around the room.

Since nearly half the meeting attendees were either having affairs with one another or contemplating them, the room quickly began breaking up into couples who seemed to be heatedly discussing their planned mergers and acquisitions. Jerry quickly looked to Susan, the sales director for the company, an attractive woman he had noticed a few weeks earlier. He noticed that she seemed to have noticed him; at least, she seemed to go out of her way to be friendly to him whenever they ran into each other.

When he looked over at Susan, he saw what appeared to be a hostile takeover from Quentin, the director of IT, who had a hand on her shoulder as she squirmed uncomfortably. Jerry quickly stepped in, pulled Quentin aside, and suggested to him that perhaps Sally from software might be more interested in his technology. Quentin pushed his thick glasses back up his nose and looked over at Sally. He first noticed her glasses but then glanced down at her mainframe and saw her enticing cleavage. Forgetting all about Susan, Quentin walked over to Sally, who shook his outstretched hand and then pushed him back onto the conference table.

Trying to be as nonchalant as he could amid the chaos, Jerry held out a hand to Susan and said, "You know, we never have been formally introduced. I'm Jerry."

Demurely holding out her hand and gently grasping Jerry's, she replied, "Hi, Jerry. I've seen you around in the office. I'm Susan."

"Since I first saw you here, I looked forward to the opportunity to working with you," Jerry replied.

"Yes, me too," she said.

Considering that Harold Bodine's assistant was currently kneeling between his legs with her mouth sliding up and down his erection and that several other couples were now already naked and merging as they spoke, the polite conversation they'd just had could have been interpreted as:

"Hey, I've seen you around. Would you like to fu—"

"I thought you'd never ask."

That said, Susan stood up and began kissing Jerry on the mouth, letting her tongue slide over his lips, inviting him to take over. Jerry slid his tongue into her mouth as he began unbuttoning her blouse, feeling her hands grasping his cock through his pants.

When the two finally pulled apart from their kiss a few moments later, they glanced around the room.

Quentin from IT was firmly docking his cock into Sally's expansion slot, feeling her software gently slide over him. She was humming like a CD drive as Quentin ran his fingers over her, pressing all her keys. Jerry could only smile, seeing how compatible these two were, a perfect integration of hardware and software.

Glancing over to the couple that had started all this, Jen and Benjamin, Jerry watched as Jen knelt between Benjamin's legs and ever so gently kissed and sucked his balls. Yes, she had definitely confirmed that he did have the balls to support her effort, and she was interested in pursuing them further. By then, even Helen, the heavyset blonde with dark roots from personnel, had joined in as she straddled Benjamin's face and quickly got very personal with him.

In the middle of the conference table, Jerry watched two accountants bumping and grinding in an inspiring 69 position atop their third-quarter spreadsheets. He had to concede that those two really knew their numbers. And speaking of numbers, it looked like Harold Bodine was locked in a long and intricate-looking daisy chain with most of the remaining staff members, and even old Rutherford had one of the college interns sitting on his lap.

With the boardroom more lively and engaged than Jerry had ever thought possible, he returned his attention to Susan. He quickly pulled off his shirt and then the rest of his clothes as he watched her lean back onto the conference table. Whatever this sales director was selling, Jerry was definitely buying, and so he moved forward and knelt between her legs. He began kissing her soft thighs, but she reached down and pulled his head up to hers. As they kissed, Jerry felt her grasp his erection and gently guide it into her.

She was wet and ready for him as he slowly slid into her, feeling her softness fold over him. Savoring the sensations of her, Jerry moved slowly, easing himself out and then back into her. He began to quicken his pace, thrusting into her and then quickly pulling out, finding a rhythm as his hips moved back and forth. He felt her begin to move with him, raising her hips up to meet each thrust. Her breathing quickened, and they were both getting closer and closer. . . .

"Ouch." Jerry felt a sudden jab in his side. He continued his thrust when he felt it again. Opening his eyes, he suddenly found himself looking at a fully clothed Susan sitting in her chair next to him. She moved her elbow and jabbed him once again. Jerry looked across the conference table and saw a fully clothed executive staff looking at him.

He glanced back to Susan as she whispered, "Your presentation? You know: 'The Company Profile Amid the Mergers and Acquisitions.'" She turned her head toward his presentation board, which was sitting on the easel behind him.

Looking back across the conference table, he said, "Ah, yes, Mergers and Acquisitions." Nodding to Harold Bodine and then to the surprisingly alert Rutherford Bodine, he went to stand up but felt a tug in his crotch. Glancing down, he saw the sizable tent his erection had made in his pants. Thinking quickly, he gently placed his folder on his lap, sat back down, and simply rolled his chair back next to the presentation board.

Reaching out, he grabbed the pointer from the easel tray and pointed to the board. Smiling confidently, he said, "I think all of us here would have to say that we had a very exciting year last year and—" Glancing over at Susan, he continued, "—I think we can look forward to an even more exciting one this year."

Looking over at Jen, Jerry said, "If you excuse my language, I must say our marketing was very ballsy, making large strides into the marketplace, and sales"—again looking at Susan—"while starting out soft, firmed up very quickly. We even made great strides in IT with the compatible software system that Sally has developed, and even accounting got together on their numbers. All in all, Mr. Bodine, I am sure you have seen the great benefits we have reaped this year. I simply can't wait to see what we have in store for next year," Jerry said, sliding his chair back to the conference table.

"As for mergers and acquisitions, I can happily say that each one of our many mergers and acquisitions was vibrant, virile, and completely satisfying."

Mr. Bodine then took over the meeting. While the company president made a few final comments to close the meeting, Jerry felt a hand on his knee. It was Susan's.

"You free for lunch today?" she asked.

Jerry nodded.

"I've just got to know what you were daydreaming about before your presentation," Susan continued.

Jerry smiled and shrugged. "I was just thinking about the

usual mergers and acquisitions, but I'll be happy to tell you about them," he said.

The meeting then broke up, but Jerry remained in his seat for a few minutes before finally getting up, grabbing his folder and presentation, and walking back to his office.

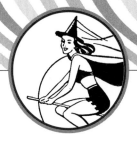

SWINGERS' HALLOWEEN MASQUERADE BALL

Frederick Goldsberry

Bright lights, big city. Gwen discovers that there is romance, sex, love, and life after marriage. She discovers the Swingers' Halloween Masquerade Ball.

The Swingers' Halloween Masquerade Ball is the best of the swingers' social dances because average people, when in costume with masks concealing their true identity, and after they have consumed a couple glasses of wine, will do things that they never dreamed they would do.

You'd be surprised what a vixen Samantha, that second-grade teacher from Boston, is when dressed as Snow White. Suddenly, she's in a circle surrounded by seven naked men, and by the look of the lengths of their aroused appendages, they are not dwarfs. You didn't know that Samantha fantasized every day for months about having sex with several men at once.

"Follow me," she says, leading them to the privacy of her hotel room.

"Hi ho, hi ho, off with Snow we go, hi ho, hi ho, hi ho, hi ho, hi ho, hi ho."

Now, surrounded by naked men with their erections out and at the ready, this is her fantasy come true. She's insatiable in her desire to get each one of them off with a hand job and/or a blowjob. Not only does she want to see their desire on their faces and in their eyes, she wants to touch, taste, and smell their desire for her. She wants to control their hunger with her body. She wants them to explode and then she wants to swallow their lust for her.

"You have a nice cock," she says, stroking him to hardness. "It's so big. I can't wait to suck it," she purrs, looking up at the naked man standing before her while stroking the man next to him. The other five men watch and eagerly await their turn with Snow White.

Soon she will return home alone with only the memory of this evening to satisfy her loneliness until the next swingers' dance, when she will return without a costume. Perhaps then she will not be as sexually adventurous and true to her fantasy, that is, until she is hidden within the privacy of her hotel room.

"Hi ho, hi ho, off we go with Snow, hi ho, hi ho, hi ho, hi ho, hi ho, hi ho."

You'd be surprised to know that the woman beneath that buxom blonde is your sweet librarian, Mary, from your hometown. She's dressed as Dorothy from *The Wizard of Oz*.

"Are you a good witch or a bad witch?" asks the blonde.

"Oh, I'm not a witch at all! I'm Dorothy from Kansas," says Mary.

Yeah, we bet you are . . . Mary, the librarian.

"Well, close your eyes, Dorothy," says the blonde. "Tap your ruby shoes together three times and think to yourself that there's no place like home, there's no place like home, there's no place like home . . . because I'm about to orgasm with you and we're both going home to Kansas."

You didn't know that Mary was bisexual. How could you? Since she was the town's respectable librarian, no one would suspect she was. You didn't know she had the hots for that blonde all night while watching her sipping wine dressed as Marilyn Monroe with her husband wearing Joe DiMaggio's old Yankees baseball uniform. You didn't know that after they go at one another, Mary and husband, the Tin Man, will retire to Marilyn Monroe's room with Joe, the Yankee Clipper, where they and their respective husbands will have a wild foursome, and we're not talking about golf or bridge.

"Batter up, Joe."

That sexy milkmaid kneeling in the corner giving that man dressed as a Hells Angel biker a blowjob is your sweet and personable school crossing guard, Kathy. Picture her in an orange safety vest and police cap holding a stop sign instead of how she looks now with her long blond braids, short skirt, and low-cut top.

"Got milk?" Or in the case of the Hells Angel, "Dude, do you want to be milked?"

She's here alone tonight without her husband, who's watching football while drinking beer before falling asleep in his recliner and thinking that she's at a Tupperware party.

"Good night, honey. Don't wait up for me. You know me with Tupperware."

"Okay, doll. I want to watch a little football before I do all those things you've been nagging me about for the past two years, such as changing the lightbulb."

You'd be surprised if I told you that Kathy will have sex with several men before she must return to her husband and uneventful life as a bored housewife and school crossing guard, that is, until the next swingers' dance at New Year's Eve, when she's coincidentally invited to yet another Tupperware party.

There in the corner dressed as Sonny and Cher are Kevin and Julie. Oh, you remember, they're at church every Sunday. She conducts Bible study class, and he collects money for the homeless.

"And the beat goes on . . . I got you, babe."

You wouldn't have recognized them had I not pointed them out. I bet you didn't know that they were swingers. I bet you didn't know that Julie loves having a much younger man join them during their most intimate moments. I bet you never would've guessed that Julie is a screamer when she climaxes and that Kevin gets off seeing his saintly wife tied to the bedposts and blindfolded and watching a young man ravish her naked body.

Here you are at your first swingers' dance, and it's the best dance of the year. It's exciting, isn't it? How do you like it so far? Are you having fun? This is the Swingers' Halloween Masquerade Ball. Go ahead, look around the huge room and admire the creative and erotic costumes. Do you see him? There on the dance floor is your mechanic from the Shell station dressed as a pirate, the perfect outfit for someone who gouges you so much to repair your car.

"Ahoy! Captain Jack!"

What about *him*? Do you recognize him? There in the middle of the dance floor is the real estate agent you worked with to buy your home, cleverly but appropriately disguised in the costume of a bank robber now that you're painfully aware of how much you overpaid for your house.

"Stick 'em up! This is a holdup!"

Look, next to him, wearing a judge's costume, is the lawyer who helped your son when he was arrested for drunk driving.

"Here comes the judge! Here comes the judge!"

Oh, and look! There's the emergency room nurse, the one who patched up your son after his accident, wearing, of all things, a nurse's costume.

"Nurse, there's something wrong with my penis. Can you blow on it and make it bigger?"

Real people like you, swingers, and you never would've guessed had you not seen them here with your own eyes. Yet relax. Don't worry. Even if they recognize you dressed as Papa Smurf covered from head to toe in blue food coloring and your wife dressed as Betty from *The Flintstones,* you're safe with their secret, too. So go ahead, enjoy yourself. Get down, get hot, get dirty, and get sexual because you're among friends—very close friends.

The Swingers' Halloween Masquerade Ball is the dance that draws the most couples. Last year, three hundred couples attended, and fifty single men and a hundred single women were allowed to participate. Preferably, the activity is geared for couples, but there are some who are looking for a third person for a threesome. Too many single men in attendance is discouraged, as they tend to get out of hand after having a few drinks and the organizers' first priority is to maintain the safety of their guests.

As a requirement of the city and enforced by the hotel, there's a policeman at the door and plenty of extra hotel security on duty so that the partygoers don't get too rowdy. It's held at a hotel, after all, and the hotel's management doesn't want naked people fornicating in the public areas, lobbies, corridors, rest rooms, and stairwells of the hotel. Further, swingers are requested to cover their scantily clad costumed bodies with a coat while walking to and from the function. The hotel doesn't want their open sexuality imposed on the other patrons of the hotel, who may not share their visually expressed opinions about open sex.

The Swingers' Halloween Masquerade Ball is a fun way to relax and spend an erotic evening. The donation at the door is $75 for a couple and $60 for single men, and single women are admitted free, for obvious reasons. There are a couple of bars at either end of the large function room that serve wine, beer, and mixed drinks and a huge buffet table that features cold and hot food. The food is included in the admission price, and the drinks are reasonably priced. Generally, men attending a swingers' dance don't drink as much as they would if they were attending a sporting event, again for obvious reasons. They don't want the alcohol to interfere with their performance later. They don't want to be embarrassed and shunned should they be remembered at the next social event.

"Oh, don't go with Joe. He drinks too much and can't maintain an erection."

Some couples attend just to watch and join in the fun of a masquerade ball but choose not to participate in any of the sexual activities and/or swinging parties that happen after the dance. Some couples attend just to get inspired for their own sexual adventures with one another in the privacy of their hotel rooms later. They get to dress up in costume without fear of someone passing judgment on them because they are inappropriately dressed. This yearly event had been happening a dozen years without G.

Her name was Gwen, but they called her G because that was the reaction men had when they saw her for the first time: "Gee, she's beautiful. Gee, she's so hot. Gee, did you see her?"

Stuck in a twenty-year marriage, Gwen was bored and wanted more. With his inattentiveness and verbal abuse, her husband had brainwashed her into thinking that she was unattractive and that no one else would want her but him. She didn't know that she was beautiful. She didn't know that she was hot. She didn't know that she was desired by men and by women. She longed for attention, affection, romance, and love. She felt trapped. She was miserably unhappy and sexually unfulfilled as a wife and as a woman. She and her husband no longer had sex because he was getting it elsewhere.

The soap operas she watched to pass the time ignited a desire in her that burned like a guiding light of what else was out there, and certainly there was another world. She tired of watching the days of her life drift away like so much sand falling through an hourglass. Definitely, she was young and restless. With only one life to live, she wanted to live it as one of the bold and beautiful.

So, much like a character on one of her soap operas on daytime television, she wanted to be romanced, lusted after, desired, and loved. Her life with a man who ignored her was a stark contrast to the lives of those who lived in her television set between 1 p.m. and 4 p.m. every weekday. As her little world turned to the edge of night, she could not wait to search for tomorrow to find out what happens to her favorite characters on *General Hospital* and to see if the women finally come together with the men they secretly love.

Then, with the advent of the Internet, the promise of a more exciting life was there, hiding in the monitor before her and waiting for her to take a step forward and grab hold of it. Suddenly, there before her eyes, were real people and not actors. Further, she could actually write to these men and they'd respond. Many of them wanted the same things she yearned to have: romance, sex, and love. The life that lived on the Internet wasn't like the life that existed only in the soap operas; this was more of a three-dimensional, interactive life. This was something tangible that she could actually participate in and make her own. This was real and this was her opportunity for happiness and fulfillment.

She emerged like a tulip in the spring. Much like Michael J. Fox's character Jamie Conway, in Jay McInerney's *Bright Lights, Big City*, who discovers that there is life without his supermodel wife, Amanda, when the smell of freshly baked bread awakened him, Gwen discovered that there was life without her husband. Tulips and bread are the best analogies to describe an image of her, something new and something familiar combined in the makeup of her renewed persona. Suddenly, she was alive again after being forsaken, dead, buried, and forgotten in a failed marriage.

G started writing to men online. They were innocent conversations at first that passed the time and made her life not only tolerable but also interesting. A dozen or so men were scattered throughout the United States, and she wrote to them. Some sent photos of themselves; some were nice, and others obscene. Like her, all were lonely. G sent them a photo of herself as a pretty girl in a plain dress. "Gee, you are pretty," they all wrote back. Weeks turned into months, and G became more risqué. She started responding to the new men who answered her with seminude and nude photos of herself. An adventure with a webcam followed. G was hooked.

Her life with her husband was now a postscript. G told everyone that she was divorced. Her husband was already gone from her mind, replaced with Tom from Connecticut, Gary from Rhode Island, Steve from New Hampshire, Jim from Maine, and Freddie.

She didn't know where Freddie was from. Although she asked, he didn't tell her. He didn't tell her much of anything that was personal to him, but oh, how she loved receiving his hot e-mails. He wrote her such passionate messages filled with humor that she wondered if he was real. She wondered if she'd ever meet him. She wondered how different and how much better her life would be with Freddie instead of with her husband, who no longer loved her.

Then she saw it, his latest e-mail, hidden among all the others but standing out like a beacon. It was the only one she opened. It was an invitation to the annual Swingers' Halloween Masquerade Ball. He's a swinger. She didn't know how she felt about that. He's been with other women. How many other women? Does he think of me as just another one of those women?

She responded to his e-mail, asking him questions. What do they do? Who attends? What should I wear? I'm so nervous. Really, no means no. If I do not want to do anything, I just have to say no.

He sent her his photo, and he was a dreamboat, tall and handsome. Now she understood why he hadn't revealed his identity to her: He lived in the next city over. All this time he was living practically next door to where she lived in misery with her husband. Oh, how cruel life is sometimes.

They met for lunch at a Chinese restaurant and hit it off so well that she accompanied him to his house, where they had hot sex, the kind of sex she hadn't had in years. If there was love at first sight, she was in love with this man. Yet he was intent on having her escort him to the Swingers' Halloween Masquerade Ball, and she questioned how he could love her and share her sexually with another. Yet he did love her.

She was a married woman, after all, and already she was cheating on her husband with this man she'd just met on the Internet. Now he wanted to introduce her to the swinging lifestyle. Suddenly, her life as a bored and unsatisfied housewife had come full circle with a dozen men who wanted to experience the sexual pleasure of her.

She dressed as a wood nymph fairy with green glitter wings, and he dressed as the boxer he once had been. They made a handsome couple and were both in demand by the other attendees at the dance. Couples appeared at their table and introduced themselves. Men asked G to dance, and women asked Freddie to dance. They had a wonderful time at the ball.

But Freddie and G were not to be. Freddie, however, was her conduit to freedom. He was her escape. He made it possible for her to consider the possibilities and to believe that she was no longer stuck.

Better to love someone than not to love and be loved. She had gone so long feeling lonely and restless, knowing there was something missing, knowing there was something better somewhere out there for her to discover. This Swingers' Halloween Masquerade Ball had opened her up and made her live her life again. Her green glitter wings were symbolic after all. She was free.

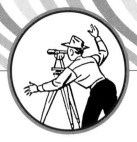

POLAR OPPOSITES

Wolf Feather

I panned the camera across the room, showing more than a dozen naked guys, plus my best friend draped across a table. I zoomed in on the naked Reiko just as Matt withdrew from her, gooey whiteness from him and others spilling out from between her legs. Slowly, I moved the camera up the Asian beauty's white-spattered body, showing Reiko in the aftermath of over two full hours of nonstop sex. She definitely looked like she had been thoroughly fucked for a long time. Reiko whimpered softly, the rise and fall of her chest drawing my attention as I zoomed in just as Derek stepped up to her, stroking himself. A few moments later, with a groan, he emptied himself, adding to the thick, drying coat of male seed on her heaving chest.

I so desperately wanted to step out from behind the camera,

to go to my former college roommate and clean her with my own tongue and then suck all that tasty fluid from deep inside her small exotic body. Or, even better, I wished that it was me on the table after more than two full hours of sex.

It took all the willpower I could muster to keep my hands on the camera, moving back down Reiko's body to show her dripping onto the tabletop. I was so incredibly wet myself just from watching that my thong was really uncomfortable, yet I tried my best to ignore it as the final guy—the party's host, my boyfriend—stepped into the view of the camera.

Seeing the very familiar erection in Randy's hand made my mouth water and caused another surge of wetness to further dampen my thong. I so wanted to drop to my knees before him and allow him to force his way into my throat as his fists tightened in my hair, holding me completely still against him as I swallowed again and again until he volleyed his love into me.

But somehow I remained behind the camera, avidly following the familiar tip as it slowly approached the well-used Asian beauty. We all knew what was coming, except for Reiko. For over an hour, her eyes had essentially been "glued" shut with a master's blindfold applied by Dave and Sean so that she could not see that her host and longtime friend was about to give her the final powerful thrills of the night.

Reiko cooed softly as she felt Randy's hand on her and then moaned loudly as he fully entered her with a single swift thrust.

"Showtime, Randy!"

"Ream 'er, Randy!"

"Make the bitch plead for mercy!"

Only Danny and Brad were newcomers to our cozy group. The rest of the guys knew all too well about Randy's extreme prowess.

As did I, which made me feel both jealous and thankful that I wasn't the "bitch" on the table, for I knew Randy's polar extremes unlike anyone else at this party.

When we are alone, Randy is almost always gentle with me. We take our time undressing each other and then sometimes spend several hours in slow, respectful foreplay. Once he finally enters me, we make love, touching, kissing, hugging, always romantic and respectful, treating each other like delicate crystalline figures on display in a museum. With his unparalleled ability to hold back his orgasm, we could be joined for several hours at a time, stopping only to shift positions on occasion.

But I also know his "evil twin" side. On these occasions, any clothing I wear is practically torn from my body. His hands maul me and his teeth devour me as if I were the captive prey of a wild beast. That is the extent of our foreplay on those occasions. Then I am forced into his desired position—spread across the bed, bent over the edge of a table, or whatever he wants from me at the moment—and he plows into me. He then royally fucks me so hard that I often sport bruises days afterward, and only a double dose of Tylenol can even begin to take the harshness away from the resultant headache, for with his incredible staying power, he can pummel my body seemingly forever before he finally explodes inside me.

The guys cheer as Reiko screams, occasionally babbling something in her native Japanese. Even a rag doll deserves better treatment. But as I know from repeated firsthand experience, the physical torment blesses the exotic beauty with sexual bliss as she surfs the orgasmic tidal waves. And I record it all.

Since I had been behind the camera all evening, I felt quite jealous that I was not the one on the table despite the brutal violence Randy was showing my former roommate.

Randy growled loudly with each violent, possessive thrust, sweat coating his skin from his furious efforts. Reiko's legs held him like a vise, threatening to never release him, while the rest of her small, delicious body was tossed around from the brutal fucking. With all the male cheers and the incessant intensity of her obviously foreign screams, anyone passing by the house probably would have assumed someone was being gang raped.

I was suddenly startled by a hand on my hip and very thankful the camera was mounted on a tripod. "You've been left out of all the fun," Reiko's fiancé, Michael, whispered in my ear as he pressed himself against my backside. His hands quickly found their way to my chest, gently massaging my hard-tipped breasts as I tried to focus on the action before me, not the action upon me.

"Let Matt take over," Michael whispered, a hand leaving me long enough to motion one of his fraternity brothers toward us. Reluctantly, I agreed and allowed Michael to lead me by the hand and take me outside.

I wore a blouse, bra, miniskirt, thong, and sandals. Michael wore nothing. As my boyfriend continued to violently force climax upon climax upon my best friend, her fiancé undressed me in the moonlight, ultimately laying me in the dewy grass.

From inside the house, the cheers and growls and screams seemed to intensify, yet my body felt like it would melt into the earth as Michael gently licked between my thighs, probing me with his fingers like an explorer entering a gold-filled cave for the first time. Michael was slow, respectful, gentle, and caring with me, the exact opposite of how Randy was treating my best friend. And while nearly a dozen voices yelled encouragement at Randy, only my soft whimpers were available to encourage Michael to continue.

But as my passion spiraled skyward, I could tell that Michael held all the encouragement he needed deep within himself. He simply wanted me to participate in the action of the evening, to take a more active role in the festivities.

Suddenly, I could no longer hear the raucous noise from inside the house. I was oblivious to the stars winking at me from the heavens. I was no longer part of the world beneath me. All I could hear were my own cries of pleasure. A billion stars formed on the inside of my eyelids. My world consisted only of two people: me and my best friend's fiancé.

After that, my memory is fuzzy. I seem to recall a tongue snaking so deeply into my mouth that I very nearly panicked. I seem to recall hearing a strained groan near my ear. I seem to recall feeling a splattering on my stomach.

All that I remember for certain is Reiko lying on me, gently kissing me as my memory became unclouded. A few of the guys knelt around me, touching us both, their congealed seed trapped between my best friend and me.

Reiko and I represented the polar opposites of the evening: many versus one, violence versus gentleness, object versus person, East versus West, Japanese versus Caucasian. I suppose the gooey white mess sandwiched between us was our equalizer. And through it all, Reiko and I had each other for comfort and support.

Such polar opposites.

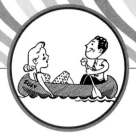

ROCKING THE BOAT

Anne Alexander

Nothing but water as far as the eye could see, and it was breathtaking. Daria took a deep breath of sea air, then a big gulp of her daiquiri. She was sure she'd need about six more of them if they were really going to do this.

She was taking another long drink from her glass when she felt David come up behind her. "Easy, baby," he said. "You don't want to pass out before the fun starts."

She turned her head to look at her husband over her shoulder. "I don't?" she asked, winking at him playfully. "I'm not so sure."

He put his hands on her waist and kissed her neck, nuzzling in and sending a shiver up her spine. "Are you having second thoughts?" he asked, serious all of a sudden.

Daria turned again and kissed David's cheek. "No, babe. Not

really. Just a little apprehensive. Liquid courage, you know." She laughed, nodding at her daiquiri.

"Right," he said, turning her around and claiming her lips with his. He kissed her softly but urgently, and his lips opened hers as his tongue made its way past her teeth and caressed her mouth. She set her glass down behind her and wrapped her arms around his strong, hard back, kneading the muscles there and moaning into his kiss.

His hands found her bottom and began to massage it gently through the light material of her skirt. He pulled back a moment and looked into her eyes. "I love you," he said.

"I love you, too," she said, grinding ever so slightly against the hardening bulge in his pants. "Hey, where are Rita and Sean?" it suddenly occurred to her to ask.

"Downstairs, getting things ready," he said, raising his eyebrows. "They sent me up to get you. Are you ready?"

Daria exhaled audibly. "Ready as I'll ever be, I suppose."

David caught her hands in his and held her gaze. "D, listen, you're allowed to change your mind about this. It's not like we signed a contract or you'll get fired if you don't. Honestly, if you want to back out, I will understand. Just tell me," he implored, looking at her intently.

He was so earnest, she giggled for a moment, but she stopped when he looked taken aback. "Honey, no, I want to. I do. Just jittery, I guess. But I'm ready," she assured him. She drained her daiquiri, and he took her hand and led her across the fly bridge to the stairs that would take them below the deck and into a fantasy. "Can we stop for a refill on the daiquiri, though?"

Fresh daiquiris in hand, David and Daria walked into the master stateroom suite downstairs. It was a beautiful yacht Rita and Sean had—Daria couldn't believe people really owned boats like this. Besides the enormous master suite, there was a big guest room, a beautiful kitchen, two heads, as she'd been told the bathrooms were called, and a massive salon. She hoped they'd get to go out on the yacht with Sean and Rita again sometime, but she supposed they ought to get through this first time and see how it went before making future plans.

"There they are!" Sean said, stretching out on the king-size bed. "Why don't you get comfortable with us down here?" He took a drink from his highball glass. Daria noticed that Rita had a glass of wine—they all needed liquid courage!

Since she didn't want to sit right down on the bed with Sean, she sank down into one of the settees along the wall, next to Rita, as David wandered around the room, looking at the framed prints of old nautical maps on the walls.

Rita looked over at Daria and saw her clutching her daiquiri glass. She reached over and pried the glass from Daria's hand and set it down. Then Rita took the other woman's hand in her own and just held it for a moment, squeezing slightly. Daria looked at Rita's face as Rita smiled at her warmly, reassuringly. She was beautiful.

That was all Daria needed, that smile, because then, suddenly, she was ready. And what she did next shocked even her. She reached up and put her hand through Rita's ginger curls and then pulled Rita to her and kissed her softly on the mouth. Rita seemed a bit surprised at first but became receptive to the kiss almost instantly, sensing Daria's need.

"Now what year is this—" David stopped as he saw his lovely wife kissing Sean's lovely wife and decided he didn't really care what year the map was from.

Sean was watching, too, transfixed as his wife moved her hand up under Daria's tank top until she found a nipple, her small breasts unfettered by a bra. Rita pinched, eliciting a gasp from Daria, who untied the cord of Rita's kimono-style blouse and watched, enraptured, as Rita's perfect breasts came into view.

Now it was David's turn to gasp as Rita's mouthwateringly large nipples taunted him from across the room. He thought he might stop breathing forever if he didn't have a taste of them immediately, so he made his way to her.

"You're beautiful," he said, dropping to his knees in front of the two women, who'd gone back to hungrily ravishing each other's mouths. "Mmmm," he murmured appreciatively as he bent his head and took one of Rita's nipples into his mouth, rolling his tongue over it until he heard her softly moan in appreciation.

Sean, who'd been enjoying the spectacle but was beginning to feel the tiniest bit left out, went to the threesome and knelt on the settee behind Daria. He reached down and pulled her tank top off, then buried his face in her neck, kissing and sucking and biting the exquisitely soft flesh he found there. His hands reached for her nipples and softly squeezed the delicate flesh.

Meanwhile, the women had gotten a bit more adventurous with each other. Rita was now rubbing the space Daria had made between her parted legs as Daria had reached down into her shorts and found her silky folds wet with desire. It was intoxicating, feeling another woman like that, knowing it was her kisses that were making Rita slippery.

"You've got me so hot," Rita breathed into Daria's ear. "Your husband, too."

Daria looked down at David, completely enthralled with Rita's breasts, which were much bigger than her own. His erection was no longer concealed within his shorts; he'd unzipped and was stroking himself openly now. As she noticed her husband's cock, she felt Sean's pressing into her back as he tickled her earlobe with his tongue and massaged her breasts expertly.

"I'm on fire, too," she whispered shyly into Rita's ear.

Rita, who was rarely shy, took this as an invitation and lifted David's face to hers, kissed him, and then knelt down in front of Daria. The redhead's eyes never left Daria's as she lifted her skirt up over her knees, parted her thighs, and began kissing the soft flesh that surrounded Daria's aching center. "Ohhhh," Daria moaned, feeling the first flicks of Rita's warm, wet tongue as she teasingly introduced herself to her vagina.

Both men sat on the bed, in unspoken agreement about not wanting to miss the beautiful sight of their wives making love. They watched eagerly as Rita ate Daria and Daria fingered her own nipples, nearly naked now. Rita must have been hitting her clitoris just right, because in only a few moments Daria was whining that she was coming. And then she did. Rita sat back, placed her fingers over Daria's clit, and stopped moving, just applying pressure, as an unbelievable orgasm ripped through

Daria's body and she yelped through it, looking completely gorgeous in her pleasure.

Just as David was about to get up to kiss her, he saw Sean get off the bed and approach Daria. "You're lovely, Daria," he said to her. "May I . . . ?"

"Of course, I —" Daria was unable to continue, still collecting herself after her explosive climax, but it was clear to David that she thought Sean was hot, too. He was tall and had a lot of hair on his chest, something David could not say about himself. He knew Sean was Daria's type and knew that she was just as interested in him as she was in his wife. Sean sat down on the settee and pulled Daria onto his lap. He kissed her softly, almost tentatively at first, but then he couldn't hold back and kissed her harder, his tongue plunging past her lips as she rocked on his lap.

"Your wife's wonderful," David heard in his ear as he felt long fingernails on the small of his back. "But you're pretty fantastic, too," Rita said, laughing huskily.

David smiled as he wrapped his arms around Rita's waist and she lowered herself down onto the bed. He kissed her lips as his hands moved immediately back to her glorious breasts.

"Thanks," he said into her ear, kissing it. "I think you're sexy as hell." He glanced over at Daria and Sean and saw his wife unbuttoning Sean's shirt as she ran her hands though his thick chest hair. They were grinding pretty hard as he sucked her tiny nipples into his mouth one by one.

"It's fun to watch, isn't it?" Rita said, getting an eyeful herself.

"It is, and it's hard to do both," David said, wanting to play with Rita but also wanting to watch his wife and Sean.

"Well, baby, there's no rush. We can take our time," she said, her hand finding his fly and pulling his still semierect dick back out of his pants. She playfully stroked it while she watched as her husband stood up and dropped his pants.

His cock was hard as he stroked it. David noted—not without a small measure of satisfaction—that Sean's penis wasn't quite as big as his own, but it was still a pretty good size. While Sean stroked himself, Daria got up on all fours on the settee. Her shyness was quickly melting away because as she positioned herself, she said to Sean, "Okay, baby, I want you inside me. Okay? Now? Okay?"

"Mm hmm," Sean muttered. He started working himself into her, moving slowly until his hips were flush with hers. Then he let out a long, low groan. "How's that? That good? Huh? You like that?"

"Yeah, yeah," Daria said, her breath getting short as Sean started really ramming into her, his hips smacking into her ass on every stroke.

David gasped as he saw his wife reach down and begin rubbing her own clitoris. Rita had chosen that moment to engulf his stiff member in her warm, moist mouth, running her tongue all the way down his shaft until it lapped at his balls. "Oh, God!" he shouted even as his wife said the same thing and then announced that she was about to reach her peak for the second time that afternoon.

"Go ahead, Daria, go ahead," Sean said, increasing the tempo again until he was moving so fast that David thought the two of them would take off from the motion.

"Oh, oh, oh, oh!" Daria moaned, exploding and falling forward onto the cushions, unable to hold herself up as she hit the peak of ecstasy.

"I can feel you coming, Daria—oh! Ohh yeah," Sean said as he emptied his load into David's wife. Daria felt it, felt each spasm of Sean's cock, and she thought it felt wonderful.

"Oh, David," she said, "it feels so good, honey. It's so good."

"I know, babe. I know," David said, so in love with his wife but having a hard time focusing on her because, he realized, he was about to lose his spunk in Rita's mouth. "Wait, Rita," he said, and she stopped. She looked up at him, lust in her eyes, questioning.

"What is it?"

"I don't want to come yet. Just hold on a minute," David begged, so close to the edge.

"Oh, I get it," Rita said, and she squeezed the base of his dick hard until he had control again. Then she climbed up onto the bed next to him and looked over at her husband as he pulled his sticky member from the skinny dark-haired woman. Daria looked like a sexy, sex-crazed mess at that point, lying down on the settee, and Rita liked it. "You look hot, Daria," Rita said to her. Daria smiled weakly, her eyes glazed. "Thanks," she whispered. "I need a rest."

"Of course you do," Sean said, dropping down next to her on the settee and giving her a soft kiss on the cheek. "Can I get you anything? A drink?"

"Some water would be great," she said, relieved that she could catch her breath for a moment. She looked at David. "I love you, babe," she mouthed to him.

"Love you, too," he said. "So much."

Rita stood up and stripped off the rest of her clothes, then lay back down on the bed, where it didn't take long for David to become transfixed by her breasts once again.

"God, you're beautiful," he told Rita, diving into her ample chest again, finding a nipple and rolling it around his mouth as he reached between her legs and found her wetter than he'd ever felt a woman before. "Wow, you're soaked," he told her.

"I know," she purred. "I've been neglected!"

"I'm deeply sorry. No more of that," he said as he began kissing his way down her belly.

As Sean came back into the room with chilled bottled water for everyone, he was treated to the sight of his gorgeous redheaded wife splayed on their bed, another man's face between her thighs. The sight caused him to go weak in the knees momentarily.

"Rita, you're amazing," he told her, handing Daria a bottle of water and sitting down to admire the view some more.

"You can say that again," David said, looking up briefly from his task before he dived in again, moving his tongue in and out of Rita's vagina a few times before traveling back up her labia to her hard button, stimulating it with his tongue. Rita squirmed and whimpered, her hands in David's hair as he brought her closer and closer to orgasm. He dragged his hand up her leg, tickling her sensitive skin before burying two of his fingers deep inside her.

David's fingers must have pushed just the right button, because she went over the edge right then, hollering his name and bucking so wildly that he could barely stay with her as she spasmed under his talented mouth.

"David! Oh, David. Oh, yes," she sighed, twirling her fingers around her nipples contentedly as she came back to earth, still shaking slightly. "I need your cock in me!" she said authoritatively, sitting up suddenly.

"Yes, absolutely," David agreed. "But I want you on top so I can fondle those perfect nipples, okay?" He lay back on the pillows, his hard dick sticking straight up out of his jeans.

Rita nodded, then pulled David's pants off and straddled him. She leaned down and licked at his nipples a moment, then sank herself right down on him. He felt himself enter her all the way in one thrust, and it was amazing. She was so tight, so warm, so wet. He wanted to tell her, but all he could say was "Ohhhhhnnnn, yes, Rita" as she began to slowly move over him.

He reached up and found a nipple with each hand, rolling them between his thumbs and forefingers and feeling like he was in heaven. She moved up and down over his cock, and on the upstroke he would feel himself move almost all the way outside her. Then she would slowly move back down his length, and it felt fantastic.

"Is it good, babe?" he heard Daria ask him. She sounded sleepy and far off, he thought.

"So good, yeah, babe, so good," he said as Rita sped up her movements. Soon she was bouncing up and down on him as he raced along to his orgasm. Suddenly he saw Sean coming toward the bed, and then he couldn't see him anymore. A moment later, he felt hot breath and a tongue around his balls, and he nearly lost it right then. But then he saw Sean's head come around as he moved his mouth to his wife's clitoris, where he spent a few seconds licking. Then he went back to David's balls, licking around until he found the tight rosebud between David's cheeks.

As Sean worked his tongue just inside the tight opening, Sean's wife was moving up and down on David's rigid member, her clitoris pressing into his pubic bone every time. Suddenly she doubled her speed, cried out once, and then came, squeezing him with her spasms as her husband's tongue found his most private spot. It all became too much for David then, and he let go inside Rita's still-shaking opening as Sean withdrew and went back to Daria.

Breathing heavily, Rita and David collapsed in a heap, enjoying the exhausted afterglow of their feverish coupling. "That was nice," David said as Rita climbed off him.

"Nice?" she said. "Nice?" And then she bit him on the shoulder.

"Ow! Okay, it was better than nice. It was swell!" he teased. She laughed.

Over on the settee, Daria leaned over and kissed Sean, tasting him thoroughly. "This is lovely, being out on a boat. I do hope you'll invite us back!" she said as they all laughed together and settled in for a delightful weekend at sea.

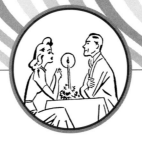

A VALENTINE EVENING
AT DEL REY

J. M. Thompson

Angela looked over the flyer she found in her desk drawer, fondly recalling the event. A Valentine Evening at Del Rey was not her first swinging experience; she and Jacob had experimented a few times with other couples in a fairly conventional swap situation. Initially, when Jacob showed her the flyer and mentioned that he had reserved a spot for them, she figured it would be just them and another couple. It was only later that she realized they would be participating in a larger group.

Remembering her excitement, she read the flyer:

DEL REY VINEYARD
A Valentine Evening at Del Rey
Dinner with Wine & Entertainment

*You are cordially invited to our popular "An Evening at Del Rey"
dinner series at Del Rey Vineyard for Valentine's Day, Saturday,
February 9, and Saturday, February 16, a four-course dinner, each
course served with a 5-oz. glass of wine. During dinner for your
listening pleasure, Wilson Fredrick will "tickle the ivories" on
our grand piano. Pick your evening and call us with a
credit card number to reserve.*

*We plan to serve the dinners in our tasting room
and we will only be able to accommodate 24 people,
so call early for reservations.*

*$170 per person, includes dinner, wine, tip, and entertainment
(extra tip optional for entertainment). Be sure to bring any
optional toys or devices you may want to share.*

Menu
*Antipasto (appetizer) —
Bacon-Wrapped Stuffed Shrimp Served
with Rosato di Sangiovese*

"Ah, the antipasto," Angela whispered to herself. The shrimp went marvelously with the Sangiovese. Angela and Jacob were sharing a table with Tawny and Ralph. Both couples were a little nervous, but with the sighs and the sights from surrounding tables and a bit of encouragement from the men, Angela and Tawny shared a toast with the wine and then shared a kiss.

The taste of the wine and Tawny's lips excited Angela, and in a moment she was pulling the woman close to her, feeling their breasts press against each other as she kneaded the tight muscles of Tawny's ass. With a quick snap behind her neck, Tawny unfastened the halter top of her dress, letting it fall away to expose her beautiful naked breasts. Cupping each in the palms of her hands, Angela lowered her mouth and sucked on the woman's nipples as elegantly as she sipped the Sangiovese.

Glancing over at the men, Angela saw that both had taken their cocks from their pants and were gently stroking them. Thinking to herself that she was glad she was a woman because she didn't need to pace herself the way the men did, she took off her dress, tossed it aside, and returned to Tawny's now naked body.

In her previous swinging experiences, she had had only a little contact with the other women, so as she positioned her head between her lover's legs and slipped her tongue into the wet opening, she was sipping this delicacy for the first time. The heady aroma and tangy taste were invigorating, and she grabbed Tawny's ass and pulled her hard against her face.

Swirling her tongue over Tawny's clit and then slipping back down to the juicy center, she wondered if she was doing it right. All she really was doing was repeating the things she'd always enjoyed having done to her.

When Tawny moaned and grabbed Angela's head, she got her answer as she slipped two fingers into the woman and felt the pulsations as Tawny came on her face. Angela left her fingers inside until the last of the pulses squeezed around her.

Feeling warm breath on her thighs, Angela opened her legs and watched as Tawny showed her appreciation. Tawny's curly blond hair flopped out over Angela's thighs as she felt the hot breath on her and then the smooth feel of a tongue slide down over her clit and dip into her. Oh, Tawny is good at this, she thought as sensations shot through her body, radiating from her clitoris. She lifted her hips and spread her legs wider, giving herself completely to the woman.

Angela glanced at Ralph and then at her husband. Both men were in agony, trying not to come but so turned on by the two women writhing in front of them. Angela then closed her eyes and simply came, pushing herself against Tawny's face, soaking it, and then leaning back on the chair to catch her breath.

"Time for the first course," one of the waiters said to them. The man then stepped over some of the other naked bodies and made his announcement several more times.

Angela leaned over and kissed Tawny on the mouth, tasting her own juices on the woman's face. She then whispered, "Thank you, Tawny, that was incredible."

"Oh, you were pretty good yourself," the sexy woman replied, smiling as she stood up and looked at the two husbands, cocks hard and ready. "Oh, you poor guys; we'll have to see if we can't get you some help this next course."

Primo (first course) —

Mixed Greens w/Pears, Goat Cheese & Roasted Walnuts
dressed in Raspberry Vinaigrette with Due Bianco

Four couples sat together for the first course, and from the look of all the men, all were successful in holding off during the appetizer. Glancing across the room, Angela spotted Tawny, who was in the midst of tasting the Due Bianco off the tip of a very large cock. Immediately grabbing the cock nearest to her, Angela knelt down with her wine and dipped the cock into the cool liquid. Noticing the man's balls tighten at the cold sensation, she quickly slipped the head into her mouth, sucking it lightly to warm it again. Only then did she back her head away, look up at the man, and say, "Hi, I'm Angela."

"I'm Bill," the man replied. "How's the wine?"

"A bit heady, but I like it," she said, dipping the cock back into the wine and then returning it to her mouth. This time she took him deep into her mouth, sucking and sliding her tongue over his head and shaft. Glancing over at her husband, she saw a small black woman running her hand up and down his shaft as her mouth bobbed quickly up and down. From the look on his face, she knew he'd be coming quickly.

Returning her attention to Bill's cock, Angela began stroking the shaft in unison with her sucking as she tickled his balls with the other hand. In just a few moments, she felt the shaft swell, but instead of letting him come in her mouth, she pulled her head back and grabbed her salad. She continued stroking his cock, directing spurt after spurt of his warm, sticky, white fluid onto the salad.

Initially Bill groaned, wanting to come in her mouth, but then, seeing it spread over Angela's salad, he smiled. After letting her squeeze the last drops onto her plate, Bill sat down next to her and watched as she ate the salad. He even let her feed him a few bites of the greens covered with his special sauce. The odd concoction was intriguing to Angela, and she made a note to try mixing some of Jacob's cum into her raspberry vinaigrette the next time she made it.

Around the room, most of the naked people were now sitting at their tables, eating the salad and sipping the Due Bianco. Angela noticed that some of the diners were drinking spritzers of the wine and special sauce. Hmm, she thought. I think I like it as salad dressing better.

Shortly, the waiter appeared and announced the main course. Checking the table numbers, Angela moved to the group around table six as her husband moved over to table five. Just before sitting down, she noted that Jacob was sitting next to Tawny and felt a jealous pang roll over her. Damn. I wanted Tawny for myself, she thought.

Secondo (main course) —

Tenderloin of Beef accompanied by Horseradish Aioli & Merlot jus
and Almond Crusted Salmon with Lemon Leek Sauce with Scalloped
Potatoes with Gruyere & Parmesan Cheese Sauce, Haricots Verts with
Roasted Garlic & Olive Oil topped with Toasted Almonds
Assortment of Signature Dinner Rolls
with Cabernet Sauvignon

Returning her attention to her table, Angela took a sip of her Cabernet as she assessed the group sitting around her. As she expected, the men were still recovering from the Primo course, so she focused on the women. Ah, yes, she thought, spotting the black woman who had been so enthusiastic with Jacob's cock. She moved closer to the woman, and holding her wine just centimeters from her almost maroon nipple, she asked, "Do you mind if I taste this from your breast?"

"Oh, my, you are direct. I like that, and yes, please taste it from anywhere on my body," the woman responded. As Angela gently dipped the nipple into her wine and began running her tongue over it, the woman continued, "I'm Altie, by the way."

Looking up at the dark black skin on Altie's face, Angela mumbled, "An . . . Angela."

She then continued licking and sucking her nipples, moving from one breast to the other, drawing each into her mouth before moving back again. She continued as she felt her partner's hands slide up her hips to her breasts. The dark hands felt warm on her pale skin, and she squeezed her body against Altie, wrapping her leg around her. She ground herself against the woman's thigh, amazed at how smooth her skin felt.

After a few more minutes grinding together, the two women moved to an open couch, noticing that all the men at their table and several men from other tables had moved with them, all transfixed by the melding of the dark black skin and the pale white. Angela noticed the men watching for only a moment because Altie immediately climbed over her, lowering herself onto her face.

Feeling Altie's tongue flick along the length of her slit, Angela burrowed her tongue past the deep pink lips into her wet center. The taste was pungent and strong, not distasteful but definitely surprising. Excited by the exotic taste, she lapped at her partner in earnest, taking in as much of her taste as she could before concentrating her attention on the clitoris.

It was difficult to concentrate, but in just moments Angela felt a flood of pleasure wash through her body and arched her back and lifted her hips, pushing herself onto Altie's face. As she came, she let her mouth slip off her lover's clit, turning to her thigh and biting her. The woman flinched but didn't pull away; instead, she simply rested her head on Angela's thigh.

Feeling a bit embarrassed about biting Altie, Angela moved her mouth back onto the wet button, determined to make up for the bite. Moving her hand up, she sucked the clit into her mouth while slipping three fingers into Altie's soft opening.

As Angela continued, Altie moaned, "More, give me more."

Pulling her fingers out, Angela curled her four fingers and her thumb and slowly pushed them into the wet opening. It was a little tight, but once she got her fingers and the back of her hand well lubricated in Altie's juices, she was actually able to make a fist and slip it into and out of her lover.

Angela heard some noise around her but wasn't sure if it was Altie moaning or the men watching. It really didn't matter, because in just a few seconds she felt Altie bucking her body above her and then felt the pulsing squeezing her hand as Altie came. When the woman finally collapsed on top of Angela, she slowly withdrew her hand, amazed at how much she had stretched to accommodate Angela's fist.

Altie remained motionless as the quivering lips slowly came back together. The two women sat up, and as Angela grabbed a towel and dried Altie's juices off her breasts, they both heard an audible whoosh as the men surrounding them finally took a breath.

One man started to applaud, but Altie spoke. "Guys, guys, let's act like you've done this before." She then looked over to Angela and silently mouthed, "DAMN," beaming, as she moved back to the table.

Angela smiled as she took her chair, grabbed her silverware, and took a bite of the steak. The rest of the guests returned to the table and quickly finished the main course.

When the waiter announced the dessert, Angela sighed, figuring the evening would end on an anticlimactic note. She quickly moved to her table and tasted the wine. "Ah, a port," she thought. "At least the wine won't be a letdown."

Dolce (dessert)—

Chocolate Almond Soufflé Torte with Raspberry Coulis
with Orange Moscato or Port Rubino

Angela took another sip of wine and looked around the room for Tawny. She heard a group of people talking, and when they dispersed and began heading back to the tables, she noticed Tawny walking toward her.

"I didn't think you were at this table," Angela said, glancing at the place cards.

"I wasn't originally, but we all decided that for dessert it would be free choice. So how's the wine? They said it would be a Port Rubino."

"The wine's good, the company's better," Angela whispered, dipping her finger into her torte and spreading the chocolate over Tawny's nipple.

"Wow, that woman you were with was something."

"Yeah, it was pretty incredible. Hey, look, she must have six guys talking to her."

"It may be just you and me, then," Tawny said, arching her back and presenting her breast to Angela.

Diving in to the treat, Angela cleaned the chocolate from Tawny's breast and then noticed a very hard and familiar-looking cock bobbing deliciously close. She looked up and said, "Bill."

"Mind if I join you ladies?" he asked.

"Not chasing after Altie over there?" Angela asked.

"I saw the show, and as far as I'm concerned, you were the

star. She simply came. Besides, I had a taste of you, and now I've come back for the rest."

"Okay, well, Bill, this is Tawny. I had a taste of her and have come back for some more, but you're free to join in."

Tawny shook his hand and then moved down to the floor, where Angela moved onto hands and knees over her. Bill sat down in the chair and sipped the port while the ladies got started.

Angela immediately slipped her tongue into Tawny, savoring the tart but mild taste. Then she moved her tongue back to Tawny's clit and ran it gently over the nub. She then felt Bill's cock as he guided it into her.

For the first time this evening, she felt the full feeling of having a cock inside her, and that sensation accompanied by Tawny's tongue on her clit was driving her wild. She would have come right away, but Tawny kept moving her mouth from her to Bill's balls and cock and then back again. Just as she got close, Tawny moved away. It was such a delightful agony.

Tawny, beneath the inspired tongue work of Angela, came first, spreading her legs wide apart. Angela shook her head back and forth, rubbing her face all over the wet lips, feeling the juices coat her face.

In response, Tawny concentrated on Angela's clit now, and Bill, getting close to coming himself, was driving his cock deep and hard into her. Once again she felt the incredible pleasure pulsate from deep inside her, quaking over her entire body. She was shaking wildly as she pulsed on Bill's cock.

Feeling Angela come, Bill let himself go, spurting deep into Angela. After the first two spurts, he pulled his cock out and let the remainder dribble into Tawny's mouth. After resting a bit on top of Tawny, breathing in the refreshing fragrance of her, Angela crawled over to the couch, sitting on the floor and leaning her back on the cushions.

Tawny grabbed a plate from the table and then sat down next to Angela. Bill joined them but sat up on the couch, letting his leg rest against Angela's shoulder. Tawny and Angela shared the chocolate almond soufflé torte with raspberry coulis as they watched the others finish their sessions and cool down.

Angela noticed that Altie was able to pare her suitors down to just two men, one of them Angela's husband. She waved as Altie held up a glass of wine and nodded her head.

Angela then looked up at Jacob as he spoke to her, "I said I still had a bottle of that wine we bought that night. Would you like some?"

"Oh, sorry, I must have drifted off for a minute," Angela replied as she folded up the flyer and returned it to her desk drawer.

"Yeah, you were long gone. I must have asked you three or four times. So would you like some wine?"

"Yes, yes, of course," she replied, watching him walk back into the kitchen. Then she shouted out to him, "Jacob, did you remember to make the Halloween reservations at Del Rey?"

Returning with two glasses of wine, he replied, "Of course, dear, I made the Halloween reservations. I know how much you love the wine there."

"Yes . . . I do love the wine," she replied, letting her mind return to that night.

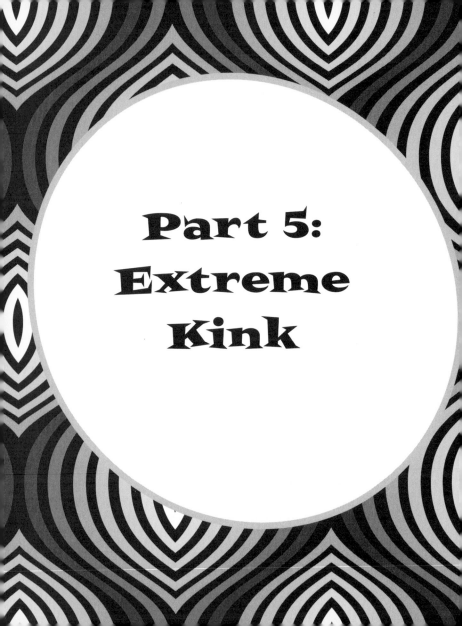

Part 5:
Extreme
Kink

Sex is as important as eating or drinking, and we ought to allow the one appetite to be satisfied with as little restraint or false modesty as the other.

—*Marquis De Sade*

E
xtreme kink? You're asking yourself right now if the two sections you just read aren't, well, extremely kinky, aren't you?

Fair enough. Swinging, swapping, and inviting guests of any kind into the sex life you share with your partner are decidedly nonvanilla activities. We've gone over those types of exploration in great detail, and now we're moving on to some other weird stuff that more or less generally goes under the heading BDSM, or bondage, discipline, sadism, and masochism . . . a compendium of other weird crap people do that falls into the category of nonvanilla sexuality.

COMMUNICATION

Bondage, discipline, sadism, masochism . . . that's a lot of words. Isn't "extreme kink" more fun? It's catchy. You can dance to it.

BDSM

You remember BDSM from Part 2, probably; however, there's dabbling in light BDSM and then there's fully embracing BDSM scenes and practices as your main sexual outlet—two very different things.

BDSM involves punishment, dominance, submission, and role playing. Most sexually adventurous people have at one time or another experienced a little light bondage, being blindfolded, dominance games, or playful spanking in bed. That's all light BDSM, and it's appealing because passivity negates expectation; that is, there's no performance anxiety. Plus, it's a little naughty, a little taboo. That sometimes turns people on.

In this section, the assumption is that you've graduated from that and are looking to expand your BDSM repertoire. But if you're just curious, you may find descriptions of BDSM scenarios interesting, at the very least.

STRETCHING THE TRUTH

This book is handy even if you are a full-fledged sex slave bound to an inversion table at this very moment. Your master can set this book up in front of you while he or she goes to get a new ball gag.

BDSM is often used as a catchall term for anything that's a little kinky or not vanilla in terms of sex play. There are arguments about every thing and every act, and some people might say that what they do is BDSM and some might say that it's not. We're not placing any value judgments on any of it by calling it BDSM or not calling it that. We're just telling you about a bunch of different sexy stuff you can do.

COMMUNICATION

If you want to call whatever it is you do BDSM, fine. If you want to call it Charles, Chaz for short, go ahead—just don't expect anyone else to know what you're talking about.

The point is that classifications are arbitrary unless you definitely need someone outside your jargon group to understand what the heck you're talking about. With that in mind, we've defined these practices and implements in accordance with the most prevalent usage. (Further exploration of several of these topics follows in this section.)

GLOSSARY OF BDSM TERMS

* **ALGOPHILIA:** A state in which one is sexually aroused by pain, whether causing or experiencing it.
* **BOTTOM:** The one who receives spankings, orders, or other types of power infliction in a dominant-submissive relationship; the opposite of top; often called "slave."
* **COLLAR:** Worn around the neck, generally by a submissive; makes attaching things such as leashes easier; often symbolic of a bond between a dominant and a submissive.
* **CONSENT:** Clear permission to engage in BDSM.
* **DOMINANT:** The one who has the power in an exchange relationship, whether it's physical or psychological.
* **EDGE PLAY:** BDSM play that involves a significant risk of getting hurt, for example, asphyxiation or fire play.

LISTEN UP, THIS IS IMPORTANT

Kinky sex is great. Kinky sex that can lead to four-alarm fires and ambulances, not so much.

* **FETISH:** A sexual attraction to an item or action that is usually not sexual; has also come to be a descriptor for all things BDSM, for example, "fetish play," "fetish party."

* **FISTING:** A practice in which an entire hand, made into a fist, is inserted into a vagina or anus.
* **FLAGELLATION:** Any kind of whipping or flogging.
* **INFANTILISM:** A role-playing game in which someone is dressed as a baby (diaper, pacifier, etc.).
* **MASOCHISM:** Being sexually excited by receiving pain; the opposite is sadism.
* **OBJECTIFICATION:** Arousal because of dehumanizing oneself or others.
* **PAIN PLAY:** Any BDSM activity involving inflicting or enduring pain.

* **RISK-AWARE CONSENSUAL KINK (RACK):** An acronym commonly used in BDSM; basically means all involved parties are participating freely and are aware of the risks of the activity.
* **SADISM:** Arousal as a result of inflicting pain on another or others; the opposite is masochism.

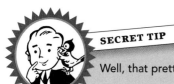

Well, that pretty much explains middle school.

* **SAFEWORD:** A word that is agreed on before BDSM activity by playmates; the word is used if things get too intense during BDSM.
* **SUBMISSIVE:** The one whose physical or psychological power is stripped in a power exchange relationship.
* **TOP:** The one who gives spankings, orders, or other power infliction; the opposite of bottom; often called "master."
* **TOTAL POWER EXCHANGE:** A relationship in which one person gives up physical and/or psychological control to another for an extended period.

FOR BDSM BEGINNERS

The world of BDSM has many practices; a lot of them have to do with power exchanges including dominance and submission, and a lot of them involve bondage and cause pain. Almost all BDSM activities require some type of role playing—there is a lot of high drama and theatricality in the BDSM world. These kinds of activities generally call for one partner to voluntarily give up control of himself or herself and be left to the devices of another person, meaning that a great deal of trust must be present in a relationship. Indeed, many BDSM enthusiasts report that this extremely high level of trust is the biggest turn-on of all.

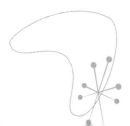

Here's another important detail: Not all—or even most—BDSM activities end with intercourse or even kissing, though they may end with orgasms. The most important part of a "session" is often setting the scene, and great care is taken to make everything match up with the fantasy, whatever that may be. As far as the turn-on: some people who enjoy BDSM talk about physical pain as though it is a wonderful, transcendent, almost holy experience. Some also say that being denied sexual release for long periods makes it that much sweeter when they finally have an orgasm. It's all a matter of personal taste.

If you are a person with a curiosity about BDSM, you probably know this already. To get started, though, you need to find a scene partner or partners. This is tricky, of course, because what you absolutely don't want is to hook up with someone who gets off on beating the crap out of you while you take it. That is *not* the essence of a BDSM relationship no matter how much it might seem like it from the outside. Ideally, you and your trusted, committed partner are finding out about all this together, exploring, taking your time, talking things out, and being very cautious.

Ours is not an ideal world, however, and the idyll is seldom the reality, so you may need to do some research to find interested parties. Your best bet is to go with trusted, established BDSM organizations or publications, of which most metropolitan areas have at least one or two.

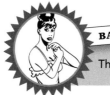
How do you find out if an organization is trustworthy? Look at things such as how long it's been in existence and how many members it has. If BDSM is what you want to get into, it's worth the time to do the research. Really read up on it online and in books (a great specialty publishing house for this type of literature is Greenery Press). Gather information before you place an ad or go to a club, and then once you do, ask questions before you get involved, or you could get hurt. There's nothing wrong with being a novice, but identify yourself as one. This is one instance in which it definitely doesn't pay to pretend to know more than you do.

One final proviso and then we'll jump right in: in all BDSM scenarios, before the power exchange takes place, it is vital that you and your partner have discussed how far it's allowed to go and set a safeword in case it gets to be too much or too painful or just too freaky. The idea of consent is taken very seriously in BDSM scenarios and culture, and you should make it a priority in your play, too.

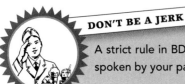

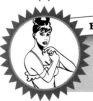

DOMINANCE AND SUBMISSION

"Dominance and submission" is the all-encompassing term for the behaviors and rituals involved in one person relinquishing control to another who asserts dominance. This power relationship may be expressed in many ways, and it needn't be—and in fact generally isn't—physical. It may occur over the telephone or through e-mails, or it may be in person; it could take place in a love relationship or between virtual strangers anonymously. It is not limited to heterosexual partnerships or homosexual ones, nor is it even limited to partnerships; polyamorous domination-submission scenarios surely exist. Dominants can be male or female; ditto with submissives.

So why on earth is this a sexually satisfying scenario that you might want to sample? Hell if we know. Seriously, though, there is a ton of research into why so many people seem to get off on this, and it all starts and ends with the fact that power struggles make up many of our day-to-day relationships and interactions, and a scenario in which there is a clear power delineation (and one that ultimately they control) is a huge stress reliever—and hence a turn-on—for lots of folks. Some studies say that especially people who wield tons of power at work, say, or even maybe in their marriages, get off on submitting to someone else in a sexual situation—thus the ability of professional dominants to make a great living and be much in demand.

SECRET TIP

Is your boss a tad too bossy? Perhaps he or she has a secret. . . . Check out the bedroom closet the next time he or she invites the department over for a barbecue.

Aficionados of D/s, as it's often known, often think the turn-on comes from the intense emotional trust and communication that happens between people in a power exchange relationship. Indeed, since power and who has it inform the dynamic in most relationships anyway, putting it right out in the open and turning it on its ear doesn't seem like such a bad idea. Or maybe it's just that humans in general like to look up to other people; hero worship is certainly not in short supply these days. But then again, neither is building someone up just to cut him or her down as soon as possible, so perhaps that's why some D/s couples switch it up. (That's literal. A "switch" is a person who'll play either role in a D/s power exchange.) Whatever the reason, the turn-on must be there for so many people to take part in this kind of relationship.

There are several different D/s "relationship models" in existence, and any of them can last for just a few hours or a day or go on indefinitely.

Generally a setup like this falls into one of these categories:

* Servitude: The submissive is the dominant's servant or slave.
* Cross-dressing: The submissive dresses as the opposite sex. (More on this later in this section.)
* Infantilism: The submissive dresses as a baby.
* Physical or verbal humiliation.
* Objectification/dehumanization: The submissive behaves like an object or animal.
* Chastity.
* Fetishes. (More on this later.)

The way you set up your fantasy-turned-reality BDSM scene is, of course, up to you and your partner and your various fantasies. A majority of D/s relationships take on the master or mistress and maidservant dynamic, in which the submissive fetches and does things for the dominant and is disciplined for misbehaving and/or becoming sexually aroused (though generally that is the point, as is the punishment part).

This brings us to bondage and discipline. But before we get to the whys and wherefores, here's the terminology for the tools.

GLOSSARY OF BDSM IMPLEMENTS

This is by no means an exhaustive list of tools used by BDSM enthusiasts, just a sampling of popular ones.

* **BALL GAG:** A ball attached to a strap; the ball is placed in the mouth, and the strap is tied or buckled around the head to gag the wearer.
* **BERKLEY HORSE:** A type of BDSM furniture used to support a person who is being flogged.

- **CAT-O'-NINE-TAILS:** A whip with nine lashes.
- **DUNGEON:** An area specifically set aside for BDSM, often equipped with any or all of the implements in this list.
- **FLOGGER:** Any of various types of tools used for beatings, such as whips, switches, and crops.
- **NIPPLE CLIP:** A clip or clamp attached to the nipple to provide stimulation with varying degrees of pressure.
- **PARACHUTE:** A device that is wrapped around the scrotum from which weights may be suspended.
- **SLEEPSACK:** Shaped like a regular sleeping bag but used to keep a person entirely immobilized in bondage games.
- **SPREADER BARS:** Used in bondage to keep the legs or arms spread wide apart; usually can be adjusted.
- **ST. ANDREW'S CROSS:** A bondage cross that is X-shaped, providing places to affix hands/wrists, feet/ankles, and waist.

STRETCHING THE TRUTH

Not sure this is what Saint Andrew had in mind while being martyred, but who knows.

YOU'RE WELCOME FOR THE TIP

Don't forget about "conventional" toys such as vibrators, dildos, and butt plugs in BDSM play—they are decidedly equal opportunity in their fun potential!

BONDAGE

Bondage is just that: being bound. More precisely (and stuffily), in BDSM it's the restraining, humiliation, discipline, and/or discomfort that come from bondage that provide sexual stimulation.

There are all kinds of ways to be bound. One kind pushes parts of the body together (such as arms or legs), and another kind forces parts of the body apart (arms and legs again). You might have your feet and hands secured to each other but not be bound to anything, or you might have chains or ropes wound around your body that aren't constricting and can be worn under clothing. Or you could be suspended from something, or your movement might be restricted in some other way. What binds you might be just another person's hands as he or she holds you down and does various things to your body or that person's voice as he or she tells you what to do. It could be a set of rules you've promised to adhere to. Being helpless is generally the turn-on here, being completely at the mercy of the person who has bound you.

There are all kinds of games you can play with bondage. Assuming your partner has consented to giving up power, you might tie him or her up and leave to go to work for the day. Your partner is immobile, waiting for you, entirely at your mercy, and you can think of him or her that way, waiting for you, all day.

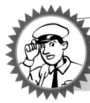

YOU'RE WELCOME FOR THE TIP

Make sure to go to the bathroom before agreeing to be bound all day.

Or you can tie your partner to the bed and do all the naughty things you've ever wanted to do but maybe weren't allowed to. Say you have a fantasy of being handcuffed to your headboard and stroked with a feather for hours, until you just can't take it anymore. Being tied up and having sex withheld could also be the punishment a dominant inflicts on a submissive in a master-slave relationship for some infraction of the rules.

The limits of imagination and desire for bondage play are the only parameters you need to stay within here. If you and your partner are on the same page, you should be able to talk it out and figure out hot scenarios featuring bondage that get you both off. There are also professional dominants whom you can pay and instruct to enact whatever fantasy you have.

DON'T BE A JERK

There are, of course, safety concerns with any bondage play. As was mentioned above, a safeword is necessary in all BDSM activities. Words such as "stop" and "no" aren't good ones because your slave will probably say them but not really mean them as part of the scene, so pick something a bit less common.

You should take these precautions:

* Don't use restraints that impair breathing, especially if you leave the submissive alone. Don't tie anything around anyone's neck.
* Try not to leave a bound person alone for very long, no longer than a few hours, certainly.

* Keep safety scissors around—the medical kind are best—so you can cut off tape or ropes if the knots don't come undone.
* Don't stay in the same position for longer than an hour without moving at least a little. It's no good if an appendage loses feeling. If that happens, move around immediately.
* Avoid liquor and drugs.
* Keep the keys to padlocks and handcuffs in accessible places, and if possible, keep a spare key.

If you're totally grossed out or confused at this point, bondage probably isn't for you and you needn't bother trying it out. But if you're intrigued or titillated, you might want to chat with your partner about it.

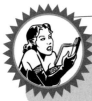

SECRETS TO MAKE YOU LOOK GOOD

Maybe read some of the stories at the end of this chapter with your partner before surprising him or her with spreader bars and a penis gag for your anniversary.

Start slowly and really talk about why you'd like to try it. If your partner is on board, fantastic. If not, try not to push it. After some time has passed, you might try a little light BDSM, as described in Part 2 of this book, and work up from there.

SADOMASOCHISM

Sadomasochism is the blanket term for the practice of inflicting or enduring pain to become sexually aroused. A sadist (from the illustrious Marquis de Sade) is one who gets off on inflicting pain, and a masochist is one who digs receiving it. S&M, as it is often known, may or may not be part of BDSM; it's not required. Often, though, it is the pain that ultimately comes from a D/s relationship—and the inflicting of discipline and punishment—that is sought. As was mentioned above, the desire to feel pain is described frequently in the BDSM community as being divine or exquisite, and it is here that pleasure is often found.

COMMUNICATION

The terms "sadist" and "masochist" are actually psychological categorizations and are not entirely accurate for describing BDSM activities, since psychologists note that a real sadist or masochist would not discuss the pain beforehand and wait for permission to indulge in the behavior. But in any case, they are the words most often used to describe this little corner of BDSM, and the suffering is real whether it's celebrated or not.

So those are the main categories of what goes in to most BDSM play. The following topics are some nonvanilla kinds of sexual expression that often go under the heading of BDSM or are included in BDSM scenes. Sometimes a dominant may "force" activities upon a submissive, and these activities may include some or all of these.

FETISHES

As was described previously, a fetish is a sexual fixation on an object, body part, or practice that generally is not associated with sex, for example feet, shoes, stockings, waste materials, and stuffed animals. This list could go on and on.

BDSM play is often fetishistic, but not always. Many who engage in it are able to get off through regular, vanilla types of sex, too.

So what causes someone to develop a fetish for, say, desk chairs? Shrinks seem to think that traumatic experiences in childhood cause them, either that or the way the brain is made up or the way a person's parents' brains are constructed. So it's nature versus nurture, and psychological treatment—even aversion therapy—doesn't often "cure" people of fetishes.

No matter what, fetishism isn't a big deal if you can come only when your man wears a tool belt in bed *and* it so happens that he gets off on wearing that very same tool belt when making love to you.

You do have some choices if your nonvanilla urges run to the fetishistic:

1. Try to ignore your fetish, hope it goes away, and try to gain sexual pleasure in other ways.
2. Talk to your partner about your interest and see if he or she is willing to indulge you.
3. Consult any one of numerous websites for personal ads and try to find a person whose fetish matches yours—the yin to your yang, so to speak.

Each of these options has its merits, and you just have to decide what you can live with and what you can't in terms of sexual satisfaction. For partners of those with a fetish, accepting the fetish is a good idea, but only as far as you're comfortable with it. If it's okay with you that your husband gets excited only when he's rubbing himself with your dirty undies, more power to you. But it probably wouldn't be okay with you if his fetish were for pregnant women and he wanted you to be constantly with child or he was going to look elsewhere, or if he wanted to have sex only when you have your period because his fetish is menstrual blood. And you might not be so open-minded if your wife's fetish revolved around pee or poop and she expected you to produce them for her sexual pleasure regardless of your feelings of revulsion. (We're not making this up; water sports and scat play, as they're known, are huge in the fetish market.)

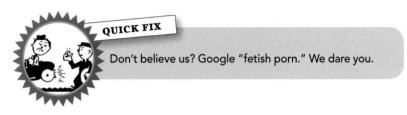

QUICK FIX

Don't believe us? Google "fetish porn." We dare you.

The list of fetishes is endless. If it exists, someone somewhere probably gets off thinking about it. There are just a few more specific fetishes we'll talk about, and they have a pretty prominent place in the world of BDSM.

Cross-dressing and Transvestism

Cross-dressing is the act of putting on clothing associated with the opposite gender in your particular culture, and in Western culture it is mostly men who dress up in traditionally female-associated garb. Transvestism basically means the same thing, though it does have homosexual connotations and is a more out-of-date term. In fact, cross-dressing men are not always or even usually gay, nor do they generally wish they were women and become transsexual down the line. This practice is often called *dressing in drag*, though that usually connotes a more open, theatrical version of the often hidden cross-dressing.

The sexual arousal part of cross-dressing comes from identifying with being a woman or from the silky feeling of women's underthings rubbing against a penis or testicles. In BDSM, cross-dressing generally involves men wearing bras, panties, stockings, and other feminine-identified sexy clothing, sometimes being called by a feminine-sounding name, and being dominated in any number of ways.

There is nothing detrimental or even particularly strange about wanting to dress in the opposite gender's traditionally accepted clothing or in being turned on because of the power (or lack thereof) that cross-dressing generates, but lots of men still hide the fact that they get off on wearing ladies' clothes. Whether this is because they worry that they will not be seen as masculine while dressed in a corset or because they have lingering shame about having been dressed as a girl while only a kid (as it turns out lots of cross-dressing men were), the shame is there either way. And as with fetishes, therapy isn't likely to help cure a man of his urge to wear dresses.

LISTEN UP, THIS IS IMPORTANT

So ladies, if you find your man in your closet wearing your nightie, try not to freak out. Or if he confides to you that he wants to wear it, definitely don't freak out; he's telling you, and that's huge for a cross-dresser.

Try to have an open, honest conversation about it and see if you can't both understand why he's doing it and how you might accept it and even perhaps be included in it in some way in the future. Outside support is available in the form of organizations such as the Society for the Second Self Inc., and of course, there are dating websites for everything under the sun, cross-dressing included.

Exhibitionism

Flashing one's naked body in public can be taken many ways, from the group of guys who run around a college campus buck naked, to the woman who gets undressed with her shades open much to the delight of the neighborhood boys, to the couple that gets off on making love in the backyard because someone could see, to the creepy guy in the raincoat who wears nothing underneath and exposes himself to children in the park. It is by turns funny, sexy, thrilling, and illegal, and it all falls under the heading of exhibitionism.

Exhibitionism is not going to a nudist event and taking off your clothes; the key element for an exhibitionist is that the place where he or she bares all is *not* a place where nudity is accepted or encouraged. That's where the thrill comes from, and that's why exhibitionism is a fetish. If being seen naked is a rush, imagine the rush an exhibitionist gets from masturbating or having sex in public.

Obviously, indecent exposure and public nudity are crimes, punishable by fines, maybe even jail time, and plenty of embarrassment.

However, in many BDSM scenarios, it is possible to set the scene to mimic an exhibitionistic display if that's what you're into, and that's really the only exhibitionism this book can sanction, even if the safe setting cuts down on the thrill.

A NOTE ON BODY MODIFICATION

Because of the exquisite pain usually involved, piercing and tattooing are often thrown into the category of BDSM. It's true that many members of the BDSM set sport full sleeves on both arms and have their septa, eyebrows, tongues, clits, penises, and whatever else pierced like crazy, but it's also true that a lot of people whose sex lives are decidedly vanilla have multiple tattoos and faces and bodies full of metal. For this reason, we're not going to take an in-depth look at this type of body modification.

Suffice it to say that if you're going to get tattooed or pierced as part of your BDSM play, do research, make sure to go to a reliable place that uses clean needles, and take care of your new adornment by disinfecting and whatever else they tell you to do at the reputable place you went to get it, because it won't be very sexy if it's oozing pus.

AND FINALLY, ICK

There's a lot of weird crap that's not just weird but revolting and not okay, and we're not going to deal with it. These are things such as necrophilia (sex with dead people), bestiality (sex with animals), pedophilia (sex with children), and other kinds of gross stuff that's against the law and against the morals of most of polite and impolite society. Even mentioning some of that junk makes us feel icky, and we hope people won't think we're condoning those behaviors. We're not. This book's philosophy on sexuality is that if everyone involved is a grown-up and can agree to these acts (not so of the dead, animals, or children) and you stay within the laws of your community, whatever you do is fine by us.

LISTEN UP, THIS IS IMPORTANT

Say it with us: there's no reason not to do whatever you want as long as no one's getting hurt who doesn't want to.

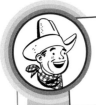

WELL, LOOK WHO FINALLY MADE THE *Rodeo*

BDSM is a catchall term to describe nonvanilla sexual acts, including bondage, domination, submission, role playing, discipline, and punishment. **POWER** is the main currency of BDSM play, and it may be wielded in any number of ways. The **SEXUAL AROUSAL** often comes from the **EXTREME** trust a person must have to willingly cede all of his or her power to another person, much as in any conventional marriage.

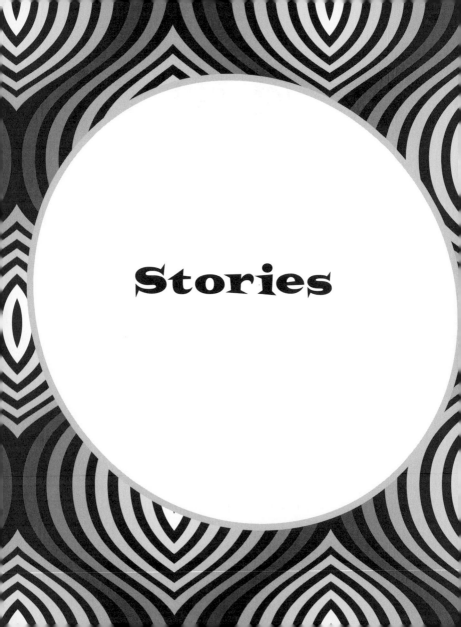

Stories

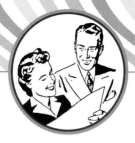

An Hour of Carnal Delight

Wolf Feather

The penis gag muffled her squeals quite effectively. That was indeed very good, since we were in a hotel room in Alabama.

Using an around-the-mattress restraining system, my slave was spread-eagle on the bed, her limbs cuffed into position. She was wonderfully naked save for the blindfold, penis gag, and collar. A sheen of sweat coated her body. Her chest had been marked rather nicely by the earlier flogging, and her breasts still bore slight indentations from the clothespins that had surrounded her nipples before the flogging.

Throughout the evening, a pair of vibrating bullets had been churning slowly inside her—just enough to keep her aroused and counteract some of the pain but clearly not enough to give her the pleasure she craved. But at last it was time to grant her that pleasure, for she had truly earned it.

Reaching between her parted thighs, I picked up the control box and slowly increased the power for one of the vibrating bullets. She sighed happily, a sound I just barely heard because of the penis gag. Then I increased the power of the second egg to match, and she whimpered around the fake phallus invading her petite mouth.

Setting the control box back to its former position, I sat on the edge of the bed, a hand gently gliding up the sweat-slickened, well-toned stomach, coming to rest on a visibly dented, well-reddened breast. I both heard and felt her slight gasp as my hand reinvigorated the latent ache of the feminine protrusion, yet the proud nipple boring into my palm clearly indicated how much she was enjoying this treatment.

"So beautiful," I whispered to her, my hand tightening the grip on her breast.

She squirmed beneath my hand, her squeals simultaneously pleading for me to release her breast and to squeeze even harder. The penis gag muffled her whines as my grip tightened to a point that I knew would hurt her even without the previously inflicted pain from the flogging and the clothespins. This was always an interesting time, watching her attempt not to breathe so that the usually instinctive subtle movement of her breasts would be negated, thus lessening the pain (or, at least, I assumed that to be her rationale) as I squeezed harder still. Yet she soon came to the point where she had to groan aloud, the sound muffled by the gag as she exhaled, her breast shifting subtly within my hand. Only then did I release my grip, noting the redness my latest action had left on her curved flesh.

I reached for the control box again and increased the power of the two vibrating bullets a little more. As expected, my loving slave moaned anew at the increased rumbling within her. Without question, despite (because of?) the pain she had endured, she was extremely aroused—that much was quite evident from the liquid desire emerging from the base of her torso.

"Calm your breathing," I instructed as I stood. I knew this would be a difficult task for her after the pain she had received, especially with the pair of bullets churning inside her, and I purposely waited until her breathing was as normal and regular as possible before moving to the foot of the bed and crawling up between her spread legs. I could hear the metal bullets vibrating inside her, constantly knocking against each other, churning softly, enticing more desire to seep from her beautiful sex.

My slave moaned aloud (albeit a muffled sound) and lurched a bit as my tongue stroked her feminine folds. Her taste was tangy, sweet, exquisite. Closing my eyes, I inhaled her scent, devoured her with my nostrils. Softly, I exhaled onto her moistened sex, the action greeted with a muffled whimper, bringing a smile to my lips.

"Do you like having the fake cock in your mouth?" I asked, and she nodded. "Do you like having the bullets banging around inside you?" I queried as I picked up the control box once more, and she nodded vigorously.

Without warning, I increased the power for both vibrating bullets, giving her the maximum amount possible. Her muffled voice suddenly did not seem quite as muffled as she cried out in reaction to the increase in pleasure.

"The slave has definitely earned a good come," I said, slipping off the bed. "Enjoy."

I made my way to the door of the hotel room. Even at that distance, I could hear the perpetual buzzing emanating from within her constantly writhing body. Purposely, I opened and closed the door to make it sound like I had left her alone, mercilessly exposed and unable to free herself . . . although I was quite certain that she would not even attempt to flee the power of the two bullets churning inside her.

The better part of an hour passed as I leaned against the wall, my arms folded across my chest, admiring her delightful show. The sight, sound, and scent of her performance were powerful, provocative. And when I at last returned to the bed and reached over her thigh to slowly turn down the power, she actually seemed thankful, as if such a lengthy period of carnal delight had nearly been too much for her.

Even after I had removed the dormant bullets and freed her from the bonds, she remained in the same position, barely moving even after I had removed the penis gag and the blindfold. Only then did I truly leave the room, getting bottled water from the vending machine in the corridor and ultimately rehydrating her.

In the morning, she was asleep in the passenger seat even before the car had reached the highway. She was so thoroughly sated and exhausted from nearly an hour of carnal delight that she was still tired some nine hours later. I looked at her for a moment and smiled, thinking to myself that I would need to exhaust her with carnal delight more often.

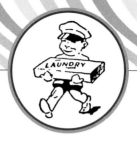

A COLLECTOR

J. M. Thompson

Jeremy pulled just past the open parking place and turned on his blinker. Putting the car in reverse, he carefully backed into the space, swinging the wheel as he cleared the car in front of him. He then put the car into drive and, straightening the wheel, pulled forward. It was quite rare to score a parking spot close to the Laundromat. He then walked around the car, opened the back door, and pulled out a bin of clothes.

Once inside, he saw that he was the only one there, so he quickly dumped his clothes into the dryer and then set his bin up on a table near it. All he had to do now was wait for the Saturday morning washers to appear. He lived about eighteen blocks away from this Laundromat, and there were probably a dozen others he could have gone to that were more convenient, but he chose this one.

There was an upscale apartment complex just across the street, one that catered to the "urban professional woman," or so the advertising said, so he figured he might enjoy the clientele at this place. Sure enough, after about a thirty-minute wait, two very attractive women walked in the door, carrying their bins of laundry. Jeremy jumped up and opened the dryer and pulled out his clothes, stacking them on the table next to his bin. He then started folding.

As the women were setting down their laundry and getting their change and detergent together, Jeremy decided he wanted a cold drink, so he headed over to the vending machine. He had to walk past both women as he went to get the drink. After putting his change in the machine and getting the drink, he slowly walked back to his clothes and dropped two items onto his stack.

Before anyone could notice, he folded a pair of his jeans and then picked up the pairs of panties he had slipped out of each woman's laundry and hid them under his pants. He continued folding, pausing only once to take out his phone, dial someone, and then hang up without talking. He fiddled with the phone a bit and then finished folding his clothes.

He walked out to his car, opened the back door, dropped the bin inside, and then walked around the car and got in. He started the engine, carefully worked his way out of the parking space, and then pulled out into the street. The drive home took about fifteen minutes with all the traffic—much too long!—but he finally made it.

Once back at his apartment, he lifted up the blue jeans and took out the two pairs of panties. He looked them over, congratulating himself for his double score today. This wasn't an easy task because the secret was to get the panties before they were washed. He could get clean panties at any time during the washing, drying, and folding the women went through, but to get the panties before washing, he had to move quickly.

He picked up his cell phone, e-mailed the two photos he had taken to himself, and then went to his computer. Pulling up the photos, he printed out a nice picture of each of the two women, and, remembering that the light pink panties went with the short Latino woman with a tight ass and small breasts and the white panties went with the blond white woman with nice big tits, he placed the photos with the matching panties.

Taking a clothespin, he attached each photo to its respective panties and then opened the top drawer of his dresser. He carefully arranged the latest items with the ten or so other pairs of panties and photos. Pausing for a moment, he grabbed the one he had gotten today from the Latino woman and then closed the drawer.

Gazing at the photo, he quickly undressed and then went into the bathroom, returning with a towel. Spreading the towel on the bed, he climbed up and leaned back against the pillows. Propping up the picture so he could look at it, he pulled the panties over his head. He looked at the picture through the leg opening of the panties and took a deep breath, taking in the scent of the woman in the photo.

Reaching down, he grabbed his cock and began stroking, all along sniffing and breathing in her scent. As his cock began to feel good from the stroking, he stuck his tongue out and, finding the bit of crusty residue left from her juices, touched his tongue to it, letting the flavor roll down his tongue. As he continued stroking and looking at the picture, he sucked the crotch of the panties into his mouth. His saliva wetted the crusted substance, and as it liquefied, he sucked it into his mouth.

The woman's flavor flooded his mouth as he stroked his cock faster and faster, finally arching his back and coming, spurting onto the towel he had spread on the bed. After milking the last drops from his cock and drying it on the towel, he pulled the panties off his head. Once again using a clothespin, he attached the panties to the picture of the Latino woman and then opened another drawer, this one containing the panties he had worn while masturbating. He dropped the panties in and slowly closed the drawer. He wondered what he was going to do for lunch.

"I think I'll try some Mexican food today," he said to himself as he picked up the towel and tossed it into the laundry hamper. "Yeah, Mexican food for sure," he repeated.

BACK TO WORK

J. M. Thompson

Going back to work after a long weekend with my mistress is a hard thing to do. After taking four days off with the holidays, this time it was even harder. At home all I have to do is put on my dress, apron, hose, and high heels and follow my mistress's instructions. Sure it hurts a bit, her slapping my balls if I fail to be ladylike, and it often is difficult to keep my bad boy under control around her, but the rewards are wonderful.

From the time I get home from work until I back out of the driveway, my life is completely in her hands. If I am good, she will reward me; if I am not good, she will punish me, which, to be perfectly honest, is also rewarding. To feel her crop redden my ass turns me on so much that I can barely keep from coming as she hits me. As she squeezes my balls, my cock gets so hard that

I nearly double over with the pain, yet knowing that sensation pleases her makes me happy.

Sadly, today was the day after Christmas, and while I had the wonderful memory of bathing her last night, I had to go off to work and face running the company, directing managers and VPs on how to do their jobs, making crucial decisions on contracts and pricing, and fighting with the accountants to try to get straight answers out of their bean-counting minds.

After shaving, I went in and selected my clothes: pinstripe, blue shirt, black belt, several ties. I was planning to let my mistress select the tie. Dark socks and black shoes would complete the uniform for the day. How I miss those high heels and that garter belt while I am sitting in endless meetings, yet in the end, it all balances out.

Walking into my mistress's room before getting dressed, I asked, "Mistress, I am about to dress for work, but can I do anything for you?"

"Well, my back is a little sore. Do you think you could give me a massage?"

"What kind of a massage do you want, mistress?"

"I'd like one of your special ones," she said, turning over and looking playfully into my eyes.

"Yes, mistress. Let me go call work and tell them I'll be late."

"Don't take too long. My back is hurting."

I slipped out of the room, grabbed my cell phone, and called my secretary. "Hey Danielle. Look, I'm going to be an hour late or so. And tell accounting to work up a draft on that Sarbanes-

Oxley thing and I'll go over it with them when I get there. Okay, see you then."

Tossing the cell phone onto the bed, I removed my clothes and paused a moment, thinking about my mistress's body, and then walked into her room, my bad boy fully hard. "Are you ready, mistress?" I asked.

"Ready and waiting," she replied.

I moved over to the bed, where she was on her stomach. Grabbing the lotion, I carefully straddled her, and though I was kneeling, I was also sitting on her lower back with my cock pressing into her rolls of skin. Pouring the lotion into my hands, I let it warm up and then began running my hands first along her shoulders and then over to her backbone and down to her ass, pressing against the muscle striations buried deep in her tissue. I continued adding lotion and rubbing her all over her back and then down her buttocks and thighs.

Working back up, I let my bad boy slide over her now slippery skin. As my hands moved over her back, pressing deep to reach the muscle, I moved my hips so my cock slid up and down the furrow between her buttocks at the base of her back. I continued the massage as I could feel the pressure building in my balls. Pleasure shot through my bad boy, and then it spurted out onto her back.

I then quickly licked it up, grabbed a towel, and wiped down her back, cleaning any excess come and lotion from it. I slid over beside her on the bed, where she gave me a kiss on the lips and said, "Be careful." I kissed her forehead and headed back into my room, quickly getting dressed.

Once dressed, I headed out to my car, started it up, and backed out of the driveway. Traffic was light since it was so close to Christmas, so I got to work faster than I had expected. I pulled into the parking lot, drove up to the space nearest the front door, the one marked CEO, and pulled in. I stepped out of my car, locked it, took a deep breath, and then walked into the building.

I walked back to my office amid a hail of "Good mornings," "How was your Christmases?" and "Boss, I think we have a problem here." I was back at work and completely in charge once again.

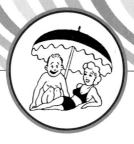

AN EARLY STROLL

Anne Alexander

The sun had just come up over the ocean, making the waves sparkle breathtakingly as they broke on the sandy shore. It was low tide, and there weren't many people on the beach yet, mostly joggers and people with dogs, but it was already getting hot.

Joel listened to the radio as he was getting dressed, feeling the sun warming his skin through the jalousie window before he saw it. He ran a comb through his dark blond hair and picked up his toothbrush.

"It's going to be another August scorcher today, folks. Temps in the high eighties, with about 70 percent humidity. Call in sick from work if you're not already on vacation—the only place to be is on the beach to get that breeze off the ocean," the deejay enthused. Joel was glad he didn't have to work until evening. It was a perfect morning for a stroll along the tide line.

He brushed his teeth as he looked in the full-length mirror and admired himself: a lightweight T-shirt, long board shorts with a button fly, and flip-flops, which he would take off as soon as he got onto the sand. He thought about bringing his iPod and then decided he didn't need it. The walk would be entertaining enough, he thought, unbuttoning his fly and heading outside.

Joel walked the three blocks to the beach quickly, excited to try out this new plan he'd worked out in the dressing room when he tried on the board shorts. As he walked up over the dunes and got his first glimpse of the dazzling ocean, his breath caught in his throat. Beautiful. Even better was that it was just as he'd expected: not too many people here so early, just a few die-hard exercise freaks, a fisherman or two, and a chair dotting the shoreline here and there. Perfect. Even an hour later in the day and it would be too crowded to pull this off.

He slipped off his flip-flops, left them by the dunes, and slowed his walk, feet digging into the soft hot sand at every step, until he got down to the hard sand in the shallow surf. He put his hands in his pockets, looked down at the crotch of his shorts, moved his hands slightly, and sure enough, there was the soft sea breeze on his cock. Ahhhhh, what a feeling. He felt the familiar stirring as he began to harden, and he shifted his hands again to close the fly of his shorts, saving himself.

He walked a block or two, feeling the cool salt water wash over his feet and the sun gathering its heat as it shone down on the nearly deserted beach. With every step, he felt his penis stiffen a little more as he eagerly anticipated what was to come. He began to walk a little more quickly, making some seagulls fly away, squawking. Their chatter broke him out of his reverie for a moment, reminding him to slow down.

Then he saw her: a girl, sitting alone. He couldn't tell how old she was from this far away, but she was wearing a one-piece bathing suit and sunglasses, and she was sitting in the hard sand, right near the water. She was writing something, it looked like, furiously scribbling in a notebook and shaking her head. As long as she wasn't too young, Joel thought, she'd be just right for him to try out the new shorts.

As he got closer, he could see the mature, feminine swell of her breasts, but still, she was young, probably in college—eighteen? Nineteen? She'd do just fine, he thought to himself as he slowed his walk even more and stuffed his hands into the pockets of his shorts.

"Hi," he said as he approached the young woman. She jumped, clearly startled at being interrupted on the beach so early, when she was obviously in the middle of something.

"Hi," she said, not overly annoyed but not welcoming either.

"Beautiful morning, huh?" he replied, thinking that if she softened to him even just a tiny bit, he'd be home free.

"It is, isn't it?" she said, allowing a little smile right at the corners of her lips.

"Mmm," Joel said, trying not to jump up and down in his

excitement, remaining in control and calm, at least for the moment. "What's that you're writing so furiously? The great American novel?"

She laughed. "Hardly. It's just my journal. I like to come down here early and just be by myself with my thoughts."

"Oh, yeah?" he said, shifting his hands ever so slightly and feeling the fly open just a hair. "Seems like you're getting some aggression out on those pages today, though."

She squinted. "Yeah, I guess a little. I'm just ready to go back to school, that's all."

He moved his fists out a wee bit more and felt the breeze on his cock, which was just about busting out of his shorts by now. "Are you in college?" he asked her, trying to keep his voice steady. She hasn't noticed yet, he thought, but that's because it's still inside the shorts. One more movement and it'll pop out. What will she do?

"Yeah," she said, pushing her sunglasses up on her head. "Home for the summer, staying with my parents for the first time in a while. It's not easy to go back, you know?"

He chuckled and then moved his hands one final time. "Yeah," he said, "I know. I've only been out of school a few years. I remember what that's like."

He could barely keep a straight face as he felt his cock bounce out into the early morning air. He was standing in front of her, and she was sitting there, looking out at the ocean, but if she shifted her gaze a little to the left, she'd see. She'd see, and then what would she do? He was positively giddy with the thrill of it.

And then she looked over. And she saw. He noticed her eyes go wide for just a second, then she looked away for an instant, then back again. Then she looked down. "But . . . but, you know. I mean, well, uh . . . it could be worse, right? I mean, uh, at least they have a house at the beach."

Oh, God, Joel thought, oh, you wonderful girl. She was pretending she didn't see. She must think I'm just a careless dresser, not a pervert. Thank God, he silently prayed. So perfect. I knew she would be. He didn't want to blow it, so he scrambled in his brain for more pleasantries, more small talk. "That's true, that's true. . . . Uh, um, when do you go back to school?"

"Oh, just a couple more weeks, actually. I'm ready," she replied, keeping it together now. She glanced back over to his crotch, saw his erection once more, and averted her gaze again, her cheeks getting pink in the ever-brightening sunlight.

She must be so embarrassed! She must be worried about being impolite! It was all Joel could do not to giggle with delight and tell her . . . tell her what? How perfectly she was playing into his scenario? How he had no intention of hurting her or even touching her? What could he possibly say? Shit, he needed to say something. He'd been silent too long.

"That's good. Oh. Well. Oh! Where do you go to school?" Brilliant. Good question. He moved his hands to open his fly a little wider, feeling the humid air on his stiff member, feeling like he could just about come from this alone.

"Oh, uh, just a little school out in the country. You've probably never heard of it; it's really small," she said, looking everywhere except at his face or his cock.

Damn! Too many questions, he thought. It's too much. Now she's nervous and thinks I'm a maniac, and there's not really anyone around . . . not even a dog walker or a speed-walking old lady. Time to wrap it up. "Well, I won't bother you anymore," Joel said, feeling his dick twitch a little, begging to be touched by more than the salty air. "You get back to your writing. I was just curious. Good luck at school."

"Uh, yeah, thanks," she muttered, already looking back down at her notebook. "Have a nice walk."

"Oh, I will. Enjoy the sun," Joel said, trying to remain collected as he strolled away.

Oh man, oh damn, that was so, so good, he thought. As soon as he was far enough away from her, he started running up to the lifeguard stand that was a few hundred yards up the beach. Thank God it was still too early for the beach patrol to be on duty! "Goddamn!" he shouted aloud as he reached the wooden boxlike structure. He sat down quickly behind it. "Goddamn!" he shouted again.

He knew he didn't have much time now, though, so he grasped his erection quickly, not even bothering to undo the top button, just stroking himself through the hole the button fly made. The hole that made my morning, he thought. But she was pretty great, too, pretty perfect, actually. Just trying to pretend it wasn't there. Just trying . . .

"Oh, uh, uh," he grunted, pulling hard on his cock, not caring that he had some sand on his hands and no lubrication, just thinking of her face as she tried not to let on, as she got more and more embarrassed.

"Yeah, yeah, yeah, oh," he whimpered, feeling that familiar feeling deep inside his balls. He thought of her face again, her cheeks getting pink as she stumbled over her words, and then he was coming all over his hand, spurt after spurt of sticky fluid. It flowed over his hand and down into the sand. "Ohhh," he moaned as the final drops leaked from his dick.

So good, he thought, making sure he didn't stain his new shorts. Great investment, these shorts, he thought as he buttoned up. He stood then, just a little shaky, and made his way back up to the dunes and his shoes and his day. It had been a very refreshing morning stroll.

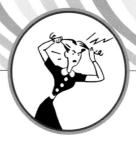

PLEASE HURT ME

Wolf Feather

We had become close friends in high school and had dated for about a year in college until we decided to set our relationship aside to focus more fully on our studies. Even after the relationship had ended, we would occasionally engage in the lovemaking or the kinky play we had discovered in college—always spontaneously, always without any strings attached. We had become, indeed, not just friends with benefits but best friends with benefits.

Our kinky play tended to focus on BDSM, almost always with me dominating her. She thoroughly enjoyed being restrained to a bed, a table, a chair, a fallen log, stakes in the ground, or anything else—any means to restrict her movement, to allow her to flail against the bonds, to struggle for freedom yet be completely unable to flee whatever I decided to bestow upon her. Although I enjoyed giving her pleasure, I especially enjoyed hurting her and over time had purchased various tools destined for her pain: several floggers, a single-tail, a large paddle, a crop, even a thin cane. I had also picked up some "everyday" items I could use to hurt her with, such as clothespins and bag clips.

When she had come by recently so that we could watch a favorite Japanese film together, the evening had begun innocently enough. Yet as the end credits for *2LDK* began to roll, she turned to me in the darkness and whispered a request:

"Please hurt me."

I was a bit surprised, especially since my mind was still filled with the unusual ending of the film. But I turned to her, using the light from the screen to gaze deep into her eyes, and found that she was sincere. She truly wanted me to hurt her, and not for the first time.

"It would be my pleasure," I responded softly, leaning toward her.

Our lips met in a gentle kiss, a counterpoint to the pain to soon be rendered and received.

In the candlelit bedroom, she stood before me, naked save for her small earrings and a slave bracelet, fully exposed to my gaze. It had been several weeks since we had last been intimate, and I still bore a slight remembrance over my left shoulder blade from where her broken fingernail has scarred me during her intense release. Yet each time I looked upon her bare body, it always felt like the first time: full of wonder, admiration, joy, desire, and trust.

"Please hurt me," she requested, her eyes expressive. "Tie me up and hurt me."

During our time as lovers, when we were first exploring BDSM, I had bought a set of foam-padded cuffs with lengthy tethers, designed to mimic those which might be found in a psychiatric hospital. After first pulling the bed away from the wall, I had her sit, her back near the headboard, cushioned by the pillows. Taking my time, I applied a cuff to each wrist, then used the tethers to secure them to the posts on either end of the headboard, giving her just enough slack to pull at her bonds without pulling her shoulders out of their sockets.

Her thighs were next, although I did not have cuffs to fit her thighs. Instead, I produced some of my old backpacking straps, intended for securing tents and sleeping bags to the backpack frame. After looping a strap around her left thigh, I ran the slack through the plastic snap closure and then tied off the end on a headboard bedpost. I performed the same feat with her right thigh; the result was a mechanism for keeping her legs spread for me as she leaned back against the pillows.

The final two padded cuffs were applied to her ankles. They had extra-long tethers, fortunately, so I was able to reach and tie the tethers around the posts at the foot of the bed. The result thwarted any attempts she might make to close her legs.

I rounded the bed several times, inspecting the security of her bonds, admiring her vulnerable position, and finally decided something more was needed. Having her lean forward as much as possible, I used two more backpacking straps, wrapping them firmly around her torso, above and below her breasts, and tying the tails together behind her. Then she leaned back against the pillows, resting comfortably.

I rounded the bed again, this time purely to admire her. She was indeed a beautiful vision of vulnerability. With her arms stretched wide and her legs parted in an unladylike manner, she was on full display for me, yet the trust was clear in her expressive eyes. Judging by the hardened points of her nipples, she was already aroused simply from being restrained.

I was already aroused just from having restrained her. I noticed her gaze drop to my jeans and her eyes sparkle appreciatively as the edges of her dainty lips curled upward.

She would soon no longer be smiling. I would make certain of that.

I moved to stand behind her, gathering her hair together and centering it so that I could massage her shoulders. Despite the somewhat taut position of her arms, I could feel her already beginning to relax.

"Please hurt me."

"Not quite yet."

"Okay."

I spent a long time massaging her shoulders, moving out along her arms to the foam-lined cuffs and returning to her shoulders again. My arousal was further steeled by these touches, by the soft sighs of contentment. How many times had I massaged her before? Yet every time still felt like the first time.

In time, I stepped away, leaving her bound on the bed. I felt her eyes upon me as I went to the closet and selected the heavy leather flogger from its hook. The many lengthy tails were indeed weighty in my hands as I hefted the source of my companion's impending pain.

I returned to the bed, holding the flogger to her lips. With the grace of an angel, she kissed the handle, then kissed each individual tail as it was held before her. As I retracted the flogger, she looked up at me expectantly, imploring me with her eyes.

I moved to stand behind her once again and placed the flogger beside her. My hands returned to the previous task of massaging her shoulders, and I felt her relax anew. After a few minutes, my hands began a slow descent down the front of her body, my fingers ultimately curling over the swell of each breast, squeezing gently, lifting each lobe and balancing its gentle weight. I continued until she was whimpering nicely, her body beginning to move sensuously against the bonds, and then retracted my hands.

Slowly, I reached for the heavy flogger. I picked it up, attuning myself to its weight in my hand, its texture against my palm and my curled fingers. I then slowly began to drag the many tails across her body, up and down her torso, along her thighs, around her neck, along her arms. She was breathing softly but a little faster, and I could easily imagine her heart rate increasing in anticipation of the impending pain.

For my part, standing behind the headboard, I was fully erect, pressing myself against the headboard for a slight relief from the growing pressure within me. Yet though I wanted to bury myself in her vulnerable body, I knew that that was not the point of the night, that I needed to fulfill my role as her caring tormenter, the one to master her.

Without warning, I spun my wrist, the tails of the flogger standing on end and splitting the air in the process. The first kiss of the leather was applied to her chest, an initial bite of light pain to her right breast. She hissed softly, stiffening, pulling slightly against her bonds.

"I like hurting you," I admitted, dragging the tails across the just-whipped swell. "I like watching you struggle and listening to your gasps and cries."

"I know," she replied quietly, relaxing into the pillows again, "and I like the pain."

Lifting the flogger away, I squeezed her right breast briefly with my left hand, slowly pulling outward until only the erect nipple was trapped between my pinching fingers. Her breath caught in her throat as I hurt her with my hand. As the flogger suddenly landed viciously between her thighs, her breath escaped as a staccato burst of sound, her body again stiffening as she instinctively pulled harder against her bonds, vainly struggling to close her thighs and protect her precious sex.

For a few seconds, flogger and hand were retracted, giving her time to drink in the pain, to revel in the experience. The flogger then befell her again, this time across both breasts, the hardest strike yet, a painful kiss that caused a painful groan to pass between her lips.

"Please hurt me," she pleaded again even as she still writhed from the latest bite of the leather.

"I will," I confirmed. "I will."

It was indeed beautiful, both visually and aurally. As I moved around the bed to various positions, the flogger tore into her, and my hands occasionally groped her violently. She was indeed a vision to behold: her eyes wild and unseeing, her mouth open wide, her hair becoming more and more disheveled, her body flailing uselessly in her bondage, her battered skin reddening in the dim candlelight. Through it all, her voice was a beautiful symphony of moans and grunts and cries and occasionally even a sharp scream.

Yet even more beautiful was the trust she had in me: trust that I would not stray beyond the boundaries within which we had played for such a long time, trust that I would not give her more pain than she could truly handle, trust that I would put her safety first and foremost no matter how outrageous our activities might become.

Standing behind her once again, I wrapped my left hand around her cheek, nudging her head over the headboard and against my chest. Tears were trickling from her eyes, and she was still whimpering from the last strike across her upper thighs. I kissed her forehead, noting the thin layer of sweat that had formed near her bangs.

"One final salvo?"

She nodded, looking up at me with tearful, unfocused eyes and a wavering smile. "Hurt me bad," she mouthed slowly to me.

In the dim candlelight, I pussy-whipped her long and hard, putting all my strength, all my desire, into each powerful strike, battering her ruthlessly, showing her no mercy. I had never seen her struggle so violently before, her entire body bucking and twisting and lurching as much as the bonds would allow. The bed protested loudly from her mindless movements, yet those sounds were greatly muted by her screams, her vocalizations of pain, of agony, of trust.

I continued to pummel her unprotected sex until I sensed she was about to use her safeword, then suddenly threw the flogger aside and leaned over the headboard, hugging her from my awkward position, caressing her, comforting her as she was consumed by the intense pain. She sobbed long and loudly, wailing her physical distress even long after she had relaxed in my hold.

Eventually, I moved around the bed, taking my time in releasing her from her all-too-willing captivity. Her body was still prominently red, especially her chest and her lower torso. Her face was still flushed and wet with her tears. Yet she was smiling weakly, thanking me with her eyes because her voice was too hoarse to speak.

I should have also thanked her, for while she had clearly needed to feel pain, I had definitely needed to grant pain, and our needs had been sated because of the solid bond of trust that linked us.

A Few Parting Words

*Sex is a game, a weapon, a toy, a joy, a trance,
an enlightenment, a loss, a hope.*

—Sallie Tisdale

You bought a book about sex, so obviously you take it seriously. Just don't take it *too* seriously, okay? I mean, unless you believe its only purpose is procreation (and again, you purchased this book, so you probably don't think it's just for making babies), sex is supposed to be a fun time had by all. So now that you've read all these descriptions of just about every conceivable sex act possible, go have sex. Enjoy it. That's what it's for.

And about the book: don't take anything in it personally or everything in it as gospel. It's a book about sex, but it's not *the* book about sex. We hope you've enjoyed it for what it is; now go enjoy the improved sex you'll have. Please.

Sources

Boston Women's Health Book Collective. *Our Bodies, Ourselves for the New Century: A Book by and for Women*, Simon & Schuster, New York, 1998.

Comfort, Alex. *The New Joy of Sex*, Pocket, New York, 1972.

Crooks, Robert, and Karla Baur. *Our Sexuality*, 6th ed., Brooks/Cole, Pacific Grove, CA, 1997.

Gould, Terry. *The Lifestyle: A Look at the Erotic Rites of Swingers*, Firefly, Ontario, 2000.

Joannides, Paul. *Guide to Getting It On*, 4th ed., Goofyfoot, Waldport, OR, 2004.

Scheiner, C. J., ed. *The Encyclopedia of Erotic Literature*, vol. 1, Barricade, New York, 1996.

Vantoch, Vicki. *The Threesome Handbook: A Practical Guide to Sleeping with Three*, Thunder's Mouth, New York, 2007.

Wiseman, Jay. *SM 101: A Realistic Introduction*, Greenery, Oakland, CA, 1998.

HBO, *Real Sex 26: "Lessons in Love and Lust,"* directed by Patti Kaplan, 2008.

The Lifestyle: Swinging in America, film, directed by David Schisgall, 2000, *www.nasca.com*.

INDEX